Gateway to Wisdom

D1596760

Gateway to Wisdom

Taoist and Buddhist Contemplative and Healing Yogas Adapted for Western Students of the Way

by
JOHN BLOFELD

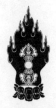

SHAMBHALA
Boulder   1980

SHAMBHALA PUBLICATIONS, INC.
1123 Spruce Street
Boulder, Colorado 80302

© 1980 George Allen & Unwin (Publishers) Ltd.

Distributed by Random House
Printed in the United States of America

LIBRARY OF CONGRESS CATALOGING IN PUBLICATION DATA

Blofeld, John Eaton Calthrope, 1913–
    Gateway to wisdom.

    Bibliography, p.
    Includes index.
    1. Meditation (Taoism) 2. Meditation (Buddhism)
3. Yoga. 4. Tao. I. Title.
BL1923.B57   294.3′4′43   79-67685
ISBN 0-87773-177-2 (Shambhala)
ISBN 0-394-73878-0 (Random House)

To Bob, before whom Airline Dragons bow;
And Ruth, to whom the Eight Immortals came;
And Al, whose skill in flying without wings
Close kinship with the Immortals doth proclaim!

Acknowledgements

For such knowledge of contemplative yoga as I may have, I am indebted to my beloved mentors of long ago – Elder Brother Tsai Ta-hai, Fifth Uncle Pun and many Chinese and Tibetan monks and laymen who most generously spent time and skill on instructing me.

For a welcome opportunity to pay an extended visit to North America, in the autumn of my life, which enabled me to assess some of the spiritual and psychological needs of Westerners in search of Eastern wisdom, I owe a great debt of gratitude to the Alan Watts Society for Comparative Philosophy (in particular, to Bob Shapiro, my indefatigable guide and mentor, and to Ruth Costello, a delightful poetess who laboured for months on arranging every detail of my complicated itinerary); to the Living Tao Foundation (especially my 'nephew', T'ai Chi Master Huang Chung-liang (Al Huang)); to the members of four growth institutes (Esalen, Cold Mountain, Oasis and Yes) and of the numerous Buddhist colleges and communities in the USA and Canada who warmly welcomed me to share in their activities; and to all the individuals who came, sometimes travelling long distances, to contribute their wisdom to my seminars.

For heart-warming hospitality, I wish to thank a few old friends and many new ones who housed and fed me, drove me about in great cities or through some 2,000 miles of fields, hills and forests, spending time, energy and money without stint on my comfort and enjoyment, and even performing such gracious offices as ironing my clothes!

May these and all beings be happy!

Contents

APPENDICES

LIST OF ILLUSTRATIONS

Foreword

All my life I have been captivated by the marvellous wisdom of China, which is largely composed of what are known collectively as the San Chiao or Three Teachings. The Chinese seldom speak of them as 'religions' because they are concerned less with dogmas and beliefs than with the art of living wisely. Confucianism, though not without religious overtones, is an ethical rather than religious system; followers of Taoism can be much taken up with religious practices or dispense with them altogether without being any the less Taoist for that. Buddhism, though it comes much nearer to being what Western people mean by a religion, is free from dogma and places emphasis on attaining a particular state of mind rather than on a body of belief. In pre-communist China, the followers of all three systems liked to speak of themselves as cultivating the Way, for the Chinese word *Tao* (the Way) was commonly used by all of them, though with differing shades of meaning. Entering upon a search for wisdom was known as *Ju Mên* (Passing through the Gateway).

With Confucianism we are not concerned here; its doctrines, though tinged with mysticism, did not give rise to yogic practices. As to the others, Buddhism is already fairly well known in the West, where it has taken firm root; whereas Taoism, except as a philosophy, is scarcely known at all. Taoist sages, always elusive, seem for the most part to have vanished from human ken since the rising of the red flood in China; even in countries adjacent to their ancient homeland – which no longer permits overt cultivation of the Way – it is rare to come upon a genuine Taoist master. In an earlier book, *The Secret and Sublime*, I speculated whimsically in the epilogue on what might have happened had some of those sages, bestriding the backs of multi-coloured dragons and *ch'i lin* (Chinese unicorns), soared through the clouds above the ocean to make a landing in the West. Little did I think while writing that epilogue that I myself would one day be carried in the belly of a huge man-made bird to the New World, where I had never yet set foot, there to hold seminars on various aspects of Chinese and Tibetan wisdom. Yet, in the summer of 1978, that was where my destiny (moulded by the determined efforts of the Alan Watts Society) took me; and I found in those far-flung lands 'beyond the Eastern Ocean's rim' a positive hunger for the wisdom so tragically rejected by China's present rulers. Of Buddhist teachers from various Asian countries I encountered many who had settled down happily in their new surroundings, though not in such numbers as to satisfy the surprisingly great demand for them. Of Taoist masters, I failed to meet even one, only some specialists in arts and sciences loosely associated with Taoism, such as I Ching divination, calligraphy, *t'ai chi* callisthenics, acupuncture and Chinese medicine.

This failure was not due to remissness on the part of myself or my hosts, for I spent more than three and a half months in North America, visiting eleven states of the USA and three Canadian provinces, always on the look out for such Taoist teachers as might be found there. From the distressingly vast city of Los Angeles, I was driven along the rugged coastline of Big Sur, thence to golden San Francisco and onwards through endless vistas of incredibly enormous trees along the coastal road to Vancouver, penetrating to the peaceful isles and mountains lying about a hundred miles to the north of that fair city. On a subsequent leg of my journey, I flew to Colorado, where my daughter, Suwimol, having spent almost all her life in Thailand's steamy plains, enjoyed walking through the snow that lies, even in August, above the tree-line in the mighty Rockies. The next halt was many-towered Chicago, whence I was driven to that part of Wisconsin where the little sisters of Lake Michigan abound. Flying thence to Toronto, I was driven through smiling fields and woods to Montreal to board a plane for Boston, where someone was waiting to drive me through New England to northern Vermont at a time when some of the maples were donning their blazing ornaments of gold and crimson to give travellers a taste of the autumn splendour yet to come. Next I was plunged into the gamut of new experiences offered by those unique cities, New York and Washington, DC, before returning to California to stay peacefully on the slopes of Mount Tamalpias, once a holy place of the American Indians. My companion on both these journeys, the indefatigable Bob Shapiro, proved himself a master of the Taoist art of cleaving his way effortlessly through obstacles; these might otherwise have proved insuperable to someone quite new to a part of the world where planes take the place of buses and a bewildering network of almost identical highways needs skilled navigation.

Mount Tamalpias retains much of its ancient magic. Though indubitably in America, it offers views lifted bodily from China's pastel-tinted Kiangsi Province and from Japan's matchless Inland Sea. Indeed, while standing on its peak, I had the joy of pointing out to one who shall always be known to me as Lady Ruth a most astounding sight: sailing towards us through the clouds and easily recognisable were the Eight Immortals from the Taoist pantheon in their ancient square-sailed junk!

Set variously amidst North America's cities, farms, forests, mountains and sea-girt islands, I came upon numbers of institutions large and small where thoughtful people are earnestly seeking remedies for the shattering environmental, psychological and spiritual problems that have arisen in the wake of the unrestrained 'progress' made by capitalistic enterprise and technological invention. Some of these, known as growth institutes, are making a broad psychological approach to the task; though by no means exclusively interested in the contributions that can be made by the teachings of Asian sages, they welcome every kind of technique for attaining a positive, well-balanced attitude to living and an unshakeable tranquillity of mind. My seminars in these places yielded a great deal of experience that has been valuable to me in writing this book. Of even greater interest in this connexion were the institutions and communities specialising in the study and practice of Buddhism. These include a number of very active Zen communities, and others under the direction of Tibetan lamas. One of these, founded by Thrungpa Rinpoche, has already blossomed into a Buddhist university; another, under Thartang Tulku, bids fair to do so; and at California's City of Ten Thousand Buddhas is a nucleus of Buddhist institutions, under the direction of the Chinese Dharma Master Hsüan Hua, from which it is intended that a university shall emerge. As to Buddhist temples, institutes and communities on a smaller scale, founded by Japanese, Tibetan, Chinese, Vietnamese and Thai monks or by native Americans, these are to be found scattered over many parts of the USA and Canada; to say nothing of small, loosely-knit Buddhist groups that meet regularly for discussion and meditation. A more or less complete list would be very long indeed, and the same is true of other institutions and groups that specialise in acupuncture, Chinese medicine and *t'ai chi* callisthenics.

All these developments are most encouraging and yet, on leaving North America, I was unable to view the whole picture I carried away with me in a spirit of unalloyed hope. I had heard from many sources of thousands of young people, driven by a great longing to discover ways of life more meaningful than those offered by a highly developed capitalist-technological society, who, being in too much of a hurry to choose well, had become the prey of gurus whose appeal is to the emotions rather than to wisdom and good sense. There had been much talk of brain-washing and even of kidnapping, of communities that demanded the handing over of private wealth and property, and of youngsters who had enrolled under one or other of these so-called gurus being threatened if they desired to withdraw. I had also read advertisements by groups claiming to teach 'tantric Buddhism' whose object was clearly to promote more exciting forms of sex! All these ills result from unrestrained, naive enthusiasm coupled with a shortage of teachers with high spiritual qualifications; the situation is all the more dangerous on account of the difficulty faced by inexperienced youngsters in distinguishing between gurus worthy and unworthy of that name. This situation is profoundly disturbing and may be very hard to remedy in a country where 'freedom of religion' is so highly respected that the law is often powerless to intervene.

My decision to write this book arose mainly from two matters that became clear to me during my seminars. First, though in North America (as in Britain) there are areas where good teachers are no longer a rarity, in others this is far from being the case; plenty of people eager to study the Way are tied by jobs or family responsibilities to places where no teaching is available. Second, there are now so many books about Eastern wisdom that people who take the trouble to attend seminars on branches of that subject are apt to be less eager for information than for instruction leading directly to *action* of some sort. They want to be taught techniques of yogic practice. Aware that beneficent and sometimes blissful experiences result from contemplative yogas regularly performed and that life thus becomes more meaningful and joyous, they long to undergo such experiences themselves. During my tour this placed me in a quandary, for spiritual practices can seldom be depended upon to produce quick results; in a seminar lasting at most eight days, even if everybody were to devote most of the time to practising meditation, notable developments would be unlikely to result. However, I did my best to introduce some action by, for example, demonstrating the ritual casting of yarrow stalks for I Ching divination; teaching participants how to chant ancient Chinese invocations and recite mantras; or giving some instruction in various forms of meditation, as well as in the employment of certain ritual actions and mudras, some of which T'ai Chi Master Huang promptly incorporated into a magically graceful ritual dance. All these attempts were enthusiastically received, but they did not (and could not) produce remarkable results in the time available. The one exercise that did lead to a sense of achievement was the practice of group healing, during which we jointly performed a type of yogic concentration for the benefit of two dangerously sick people, whose subsequent recovery was so rapid as to make it seem very likely that the practice had been effective. This encouraged me to consider writing a book on simple yogas that could guide people to similarly effective action, if designed specifically to meet the needs of Westerners under the circumstances now prevailing in North America and Europe.

When the idea first occurred to me, I hesitated. The attainment of expanded states of consciousness during which exalted spiritual insights are experienced demands not only sustained and rigorous practice, but also accurate knowledge and strict discipline of mind and body. Hence, the personal supervision and guidance of a teacher are highly desirable; without such aid, things may go seriously wrong. On this account, I put the thought away for a time, but it kept recurring.

'Even the longest journey must begin with a single step', as the Chinese saying goes. One can, as I know from experience, go at least a short way towards a high yogic goal while progressing on one's own. This being so, I realised that there is room for a book that could be used at the initial stages of the path in preparation for a time when the opportunity arises to acquire the personal guidance of a well qualified teacher. The reader should clearly understand that a mere book can – except in very rare cases – take him only a little of the way. By following some of the yogic practices described in the following pages and developing the necessary attitude towards them, he can, however, begin to enhance the quality of life for himself and those around him, besides preparing for the day when a teacher becomes available. Yet it would be reckless for him to think of proceeding to those wider seas where fierce currents and submerged rocks imperil all who sail there without the assistance of a pilot who knows how to find his way past those dangerous obstacles. The book may also be of some use to those people who have been set on the right path by a good teacher, but whose circumstances do not permit them to remain within reach of him – a situation in which I have often found myself. For them, some of the practices set forth here may prove useful auxiliaries to whatever main practice they have, perforce, but incompletely mastered.

The aims, then, of this book are:
 to enhance the quality of life in the Here and Now through realisation of the essential holiness and underlying unity of oneself, all living beings and the whole environment;
 to inculcate some of the attitudes required for more meaningful living, and in preparation for setting out upon a course for Enlightenment (though no attempt has been made to chart the further stages of that course, for which a teacher's supervision is an absolute requirement).

These aims involve:
   *achieving some notion of the nature of reality as perceived by mystics in
exalted states of expanded consciousness, this knowledge being fundamental to all yogic attainment;*
   understanding why the entire universe is to be revered as holy;
   cultivating man's lost sense of awe;
   *recognising that the development of wisdom and compassion must go
hand in hand;*
   transmutation of negative emotions and inordinate desires;
   *attaining inner stillness and a state of tranquillity invulnerable to life's
ups and downs.*

Yogic means of accomplishing them comprise:
   fostering simplicity and frugality;
   contemplative attunement to nature's rhythms;
   contemplative examination of the nature of 'self' and 'other';
   the practice of awareness;
   various meditative techniques;
   the practice of individual and group healing;
   *such aids to progress as yogic breathing and exercises, chants, mantras,
mudras, creative arts, regulation of diet and sexual intercourse, etc.*

These matters are not dealt with in a particular order; some receive
lengthy treatment, others are merely touched upon, for they impinge
upon one another and whereas some require rigorous practice others
arise of themselves as the fruits of progress. Nor does the book run
smoothly from shallow into deeper waters; on the contrary, the most
profound teachings occur in the introductory sections to each of the
book's main parts. This is because, although the actual practices are
simple, the theory underlying them is the same as for highly advanced
yogas. The simplicity of the practices is, moreover, in some cases
more apparent than real; most can be raised to increasingly lofty levels
of performance, their content deepening as they are pursued. It is not
intended that any reader should undertake all the practices; each will
require a good deal of time to become thoroughly effective. (For
example, one can learn to recite a short mantra in a minute or so, but
its effectiveness will depend on 'mastering it', which requires frequent recitation over a long period.) The exposition with which each
of the parts, Taoist and Buddhist, begins has been kept to a bare
minimum; therefore it requires careful study as this knowledge is
essential to the proper performance of the yogas; for whatever has to
be done with body, hands or tongue owes its importance solely (or

very largely) to its effect upon the mind. Mind is pre-eminent. Mind is the king.

My use of the term 'yoga', and also of 'yogin' for one who practises contemplation, may require explanation. 'Yoga' is cognate with the English words 'union' and 'unite'; it was originally employed in India in the sense of 'union with God' and extended to cover the various spiritual exercises practised to this end. Unfortunately it has passed into the English language at the popular level as a synonym for *hatha yoga*, which connotes just the *physical* exercises related to yoga as a whole, with the result that misunderstanding of its full meaning has arisen. 'Yoga' is used in this book neither in its ancient Hindu nor in its popular English sense. Since Taoists and Buddhists do not believe in a personal Creator, they never seek to attain union with God. They hold that all beings are fundamentally indivisible from (and therefore do not require to be united with) the ground of being, from which man feels himself to be separate only on account of faulty perception. From this faulty perception arises the need for what Taoists term 'Return to the Source' and Buddhists call 'Enlightenment' – a transcendental experience that sunders the bonds of ego-delusion. The experience is accompanied by sensations of blissfulness and hitherto unimaginable freedom. It consists not in attaining unity with the ground of being, since that has never been interrupted, but of joyous perception of that unity, to which they have long been blind. In this context, 'yoga' means *full realisation of an already existing but hitherto unperceived state of union*; by extension it also connotes the various means of attaining this supreme intuitive experience. A yogin is one who employs such means, whether to reach Enlightenment or to achieve more limited objectives along the Way that will raise his potentiality for intuitive experiences and meanwhile reconcile him joyously with his environment. Since his mind is the source of all high endeavour and the receptacle of all deeply meaningful experience, essential yogic practice has far more to do with mind than body (although the well-being of the body is certainly not to be neglected). Therefore, yogic practices are mainly mental in character, there being, by the way, no distinction in this terminology between mind and spirit. I myself sometimes employ the word 'spiritual' because of its inspiring connotations in our language, but my use of it is wholly rhetorical. Indeed, in an ultimate sense, even the distinction between mind and body is found by yogins to be invalid.

In general, I have closely followed Taoist and Mahayana Buddhist tradition, but made some modifications to suit what I deem to be Western needs. In transplanting a tradition from one culture to another, one should not be too particular about detail, but take great care to retain the essence in unchanged form. Taoism, unlike Buddhism, has hitherto been confined to its native country, whence it has been swept away by the coming of the red tide, so there is no satisfactory way of obtaining guidance as to what degrees of adaptation will enable it to flourish on new soil. Buddhism has, from very early times, freely adapted itself to the cultures of different countries, taking on much local colour wherever it has spread, yet without diluting its essence or losing its essential flavour; so its further adaptation fully accords with precedent. Unfortunately, in going about the task, I have been unable to attain sanction from my Chinese teachers, having lost all contact with any of them who may survive; nor is it likely that they are still in this world, for they would now be immensely old. Therefore the responsibility rests with me alone – a responsibility I should have been loath to take but for the fact that the practices concerned do not involve the manipulation of powerful energies (other than the *mahā karunā* of the compassionate Kuan Yin Bodhisattva) and are not at all likely to do damage to those who undertake them without a teacher. Even so, I ask pardon from my teachers and guardian deities for any errors that may have crept in.

I have been a little tempted to write this book under my Taoist name, Niu-t'ou Tao-jên (the Oxhead Recluse), chosen partly on account of my birth-year and partly because my head is unusually large. Like many Taoist cognomens, it is a fun-name. But it would not do at all to delude any readers into supposing it to be the work of a genuine Chinese sage, for the difference between one who has absorbed Chinese wisdom with his mother's milk and one who has stumbled upon facets of it in a desultory way is very great.

John Blofeld

Written in Wu Wei Studio (a place where things may be allowed to happen of themselves), spring, the Year of the Sheep (1979).

Part I *Taoist Theory and Practice*

A THEORY

1

Nature's Grand Design

The Taoist concept of the nature of the universe agrees closely with the Buddhist concept (set forth in part II). It is at once so utterly sublime and so extraordinarily up to date that modern physicists have only recently begun to feel their way towards accepting the same general principle. In this concept, the notion of an omnipotent creator-deity separate from his creation plays no part at all. Belief in God gives place to reverential awe for the majesty and mystery of the cosmos itself. Taoist sages have never presumed to define the ultimate; for, as the great Lao-tzû asserts in the *Tao Tê Ching* written two and a half millennia ago, 'He who speaks [of the Tao] does not know; he who knows does not speak'. He also writes: 'The Tao expressible in words is not the eternal Tao; a name that can be spoken is not that of the eternal Tao.' By the Tao (literally 'the Way') he refers not to a power standing outside phenomena, but to the very substance – or, better, non-substance – of the universe. As accomplished mystics belonging to many diverse cultures have come to realise from the direct confrontation with reality that forms the very apex of mystical experience, the supremely holy creative principle is not a *being* to be loved or placated by hymns and sacrifice, but rather a *state of being* that is manifest throughout the cosmos and lies apart from nothing, since it is the very essence of all existence.

The sublime Tao is that which lies right in front of (and equally in and behind) our eyes. Far from being apart from it, as souls according to Christian theology are apart from God, we are permeated by it and partake of its very being. That most of us experience a sense of loneliness, of apartness both from the highest reality and from all the beings and objects around us, is due to deluded understanding and a faulty sense perception, which lead us to think in terms of 'I am I; other is other'. Yet so deep-seated is this delusion that even Taoist yogins speak of the supreme mystical apotheosis at which they aim as

'Return to the Source'; nevertheless, they are aware that this is a misnomer, for one cannot *return* to that from which no one has ever for one instant been apart. 'Return to the Source' is a figurative term for the unutterably blissful experience of *becoming aware with all one's being* of perfect identity with all that is, has been or ever could be.

People with a Christian or Jewish background are apt to suppose that absence of belief in an omnipotent creator-deity necessarily implies acceptance of the doctrine of materialism. This, however, is a great error. A Taoist would be better pleased if you were to describe him as a follower of the doctrine that matter is essentially spirit; for, though in fact his thought penetrates beyond such distinctions, his concept of the cosmos comes very much closer to that of an unblemished spiritual whole than to what is commonly implied by the doctrine of materialism. He recognises both spirit and matter to be indivisible manifestations of the formless, measureless, ever-existing, undifferentiated and essentially unchanging Tao, properly called the Nameless because beyond description, but arbitrarily named the Way for the sake of convenience. The Tao is the Way, but also the Source, the Journey, the Traveller and the Goal. One may choose to conceive of it as matter or spirit, or as both of these or neither; such distinctions are valid only for as long as we remain at a very imperfect level of consciousness. Nothing is so poor or insignificant as to be other in nature than all that is most glorious and profound; therefore, even the most ordinary people, animals and things are worthy of the utmost reverence. A man, his fellow men, all sentient beings, their environment and the entire cosmos are inextricably bound together; all alike are tangible but purely transient manifestations of intangible, undifferentiated, illimitable, timeless being – the Tao. In bowing to you, I bow to one greater than God. In inhaling the scent of a rose or the stink of dung, I am breathing in the very essence of being; to admire the one and feel disgusted by the other is to make a worthless and even harmful distinction. The Taoist sage is one who has learnt to cherish every corner, every atom of the environment, to avoid unnecessary interference even with the tiniest or most repulsive of creatures. Ants and cockroaches, no less than man, are manifestations of the Tao; they, too, have their place, their right to cling to life, their aversion to pain and hunger, their need to escape these evils by the means natural to their species. Man is not the lord of the universe; he is doomed to perish if he flies for long in the face of nature and, should that happen, the ants and cockroaches will not even be aware of his demise. Arrogance has no place in Taoism.

Another error likely to arise in the minds of people only superficially acquainted with Taoism stems from the blending that has taken place between that enlightened philosophy and the ancient Chinese folk religion. Some, though by no means all, Taoists go along with that ancient faith in peopling the universe with divers orders of supernatural beings. This notion is sometimes confused with theism and has also led to the supposition that Taoism is a rather primitive system of belief. The notion is, however, by no means central to Taoism; one may accept or reject it without thereby becoming any more or any less a Taoist. In any case, it has nothing to do with a theistic concept of the universe; for gods and demons are recognised by those who credit their existence as part of the universal order, as transient manifestations of the Tao not essentially different from tangible orders of being, such as people, animals and plants, and therefore subject to birth, growth, decay and dissolution like all the rest. Just as elephants have longer lives than mayflies, so may gods live much longer than humans and have special powers and characteristics belonging to their species; but in no sense are they above the universe or empowered to modify the overall workings of the Tao. To use familiar Christian terminology, they are creatures; not one of them can be identified with a creator-deity.

Belief in a multitude of gods and demons is widely regarded by modern man as a characteristic of the more primitive forms of religion, but this attitude demands further examination. Until recently at least, people all over the world, whatever their cultures and creeds, felt sensible of the presence of unseen powers, benificent and baleful. Were they altogether wrong? I myself would hesitate to assert that there can be no such beings as gods and demons, angels or whatever. It depends on how one views them. One sees crowds swayed by forces alien to the individuals who compose them, and one knows from experience that a person is sometimes mastered by an overwhelming impulse quite contrary to his nature. It is common to encounter instances of what seem very much like the operation of spells of good luck or misfortune. There are certain mental states that at least have the appearance of spirit possession. Then, again, everyone who regularly practises contemplative yoga (meditation as it is now rather incorrectly called) becomes aware of hitherto unsuspected forces that, rising in the mind, threaten further progress by destroying the yogin's hard-won tranquillity and making concentration wellnigh impossible at times; and there are other times when it seems that sweetly benign forces are assisting him smoothly forward towards his goal. What exactly are all the forces involved in these various instances? Modern man has names for them, but he can seldom provide more than tentative explanations, and learned names are often used to conceal lack of comprehension. Are these forces internal or external, or both? Conceiving of some of them in the form of demons with fiery eyes and pointed fangs may strike us as laughably out of step with the spirit of the age, yet psychic phenomena of all kinds are less frequently laughed at than was the case just a few years ago. Of chief consequence is the fact that impulses not consonant with a person's character do arise, and that sometimes they overwhelm him and cause great havoc. Whether one thinks of them as demons or psychoses, the effects are there for all to see, and I have known some of them to be cured by methods evolved for the subjugation of demons. The different names and interpretations given to them are matters of cultural background; to dismiss them as non-existent is patently absurd. All that matters is that they should be effectively dealt with, and Taoists strike me as often being better equipped to do that than a good many psychiatrists, which makes the word 'primitive' in this connexion seem inept.

In any case, in performing contemplative yoga one has to reckon with mysterious forces, whatever their origin may be; but I hope I have made it clear that the whole realm of psychic phenomena is merely incidental to (and quite often absent from) the grand Taoist concept of existence. Of much greater consequence is the point made earlier that the real enemies of yogic progress are not demons but man's own propensity to make false distinctions, clinging to this, abhorring that, reverencing spirit, despising matter (or the reverse), loving self and being indifferent to or hating other. Until these distinctions are overcome, progress is bound to be slow; whereas in the blissful experience, Return to the Source, all notion of I and other is utterly dissolved.

2

Some Taoist
Concepts

(a) NO DUALITY

In the *Tao Tê Ching* it is written: 'The cosmos originated in what may be called the mother of heaven and earth. To grasp the mother is to come to know the child; to know the child is to hold fast to the mother and life becomes secure.' 'Mother' has no anthropomorphic signification here; it just means the formless aspect of the Tao, which closely corresponds to the Buddhist *śunyata* or void, and signifies the cosmos viewed as an undifferentiated unity. ⌜Son⌝, on the other hand, connotes the cosmos viewed as a multitude of shifting forms. To perceive and understand the one is to comprehend the true nature of the other, and vice versa. To neglect the mother is to cling to material things and be lost to a sense of mystery and awe, to judge life by mere appearances. To neglect the child is to despise the material world and suppose that true beauty and goodness are to be found elsewhere – the error of the medieval Christians. Beauty, goodness and meaning are to be found right here before our eyes. Our failure to perceive them lies in our own faulty perception, not in the nature of life itself. Spirit and matter are one; here and beyond are one; full perception of this arises with the dawning of inner stillness during contemplative yoga.

In the *Tao Tê Ching* it is also written: 'IS NOT is the name of the beginning of the cosmos. IS is the name of the matrix of the myriad objects.' The sage goes on to say that, when one desires to view the mystery of existence as a whole, the mind concentrates on IS NOT, the limitless, intangible, undifferentiated non-substance of the Tao; whereas, when one desires to view the fringes of reality (as do scientists when concentrating on any particular principle, law or phenomenon), the mind concentrates on IS. But, as Lao-tzû tells us, 'these two spring from a common source, though differently named. Both are called mysterious. Mystery upon mystery, the gateway to all marvels.' This passage at once brings to mind the Buddhist teaching 'form is void; void is form'; phrased in familiar Western terms, it means (among other things) that matter is spirit; spirit, matter. The Tao is at once the seemless, intangible void *and* all that confronts us in the Here and Now apparent to our senses. These are NOT TWO!

(b) *YIN* AND *YANG*

The *Tao Tê Ching*, in asserting elsewhere that 'the one becomes two', signifies the manner in which the intangible Tao manifests itself as a cosmos containing myriads of shifting forms through the operation of the principle of polarity, the interaction of the polar forces *yin* and *yang*. *Yin*, primarily meaning the sunless side of a mountain, signifies the receptive aspect of phenomena; *yang*, the mountain's sunny side, signifies their dynamic aspect. These must not be regarded as opposites, but clearly recognised as 'two sides of the same coin', for neither could exist in the absence of the other. There could be no light without dark, no dynamism without stillness, no plus without minus, no doing without done-to. Nor must one suppose *yin* to be inferior to *yang*. There could be no procreation without female, no hills without valleys, no burgeoning of plants without subsequent ripeness and decay. *Yin* and *yang* are present in all conceivable phenomena, and not to be found in isolation from each other, for pure *yang* contains the seed of *yin*, pure *yin* contains the seed of *yang*, as exemplified by the female characteristics to be found in every male and vice versa. It is through varying interactions of *yin* and *yang* that phenomena come to differ from one another; when the *yin* and *yang* components of a phenomenon cease to dwell in harmony, it thereupon disintegrates; and, with renewal of their harmonious interaction, something else comes into being. Philosophically this interplay has an important lesson for the yogic adept, whose ever-deepening intuitive perception leads him to accept with smiling equanimity ups and downs, gains and losses, growth and decay, life and death.

(c) PERPETUAL CHANGE

The one unchanging factor in the cosmos is change itself. Nothing remains the same even for an instant, yet this by no means results in a chaotic state of uncontrolled flux. The transformations of the Tao follow regular cyclic patterns, exemplified by the orbits of heavenly bodies, the progression of the seasons, the alternation of night and day, the sequence of birth, growth, decay and dissolution through which everything must pass. Yet the ever-changing remains forever unchanged. The cosmic non-substance of the Tao is not subject to augmentation or decrease; what is more, as the American thinker Emerson intuited, the infinite ocean of being has the mysterious property of being wholly present in the smallest imaginable entity. The non-substance of the Tao resembles pure consciousness in not being governed by the laws of space.

Though awesomely holy, the Tao does not require worship, being unaffected by praise or blame. In the words of the *Tao Tê Ching*, 'the myriad objects owe their existence to the Tao, but it claims no lordship; it accomplishes all, yet does not seek to possess'. It is proper to view the self-existent cosmos and its majestic changes and transformations with reverence and awe, but to compose prayers or hymns to it would be merely futile. The Tao is not concerned with the rise or fall of individuals, but with the smooth effortless progress of its transformations, the well-being of the whole. Therefore the yogic adept achieves his goal not by imploring the Tao to favour him but by learning to accommodate himself to its harmonious workings.

(d) THE FIVE ACTIVITIES (*WU HSING*)

The play of perpetual orderly change is a subject that seems to have entranced early Taoists with scientific leanings, of whom there were many. They sought to analyse, and thereby be able to forecast, the interactions of nature's forces, in terms not only of *yin–yang* polarity, but also of five broad categories of mutually supportive and mutually destructive activity. Unfortunately, the names given to these five – metal, wood, water, fire and earth – are so reminiscent of those of the four elements in the ancient Greek cosmology that the term *wu hsing* has often been incorrectly translated 'the five elements', although the Chinese syllables clearly mean 'the five activities', for *wu* means 'five' and *hsing* has the basic meaning of 'to walk, to act, to do'. Elements are static, *hsing* dynamic.

Metal signifies activities involving strength, endurance, resistance, delay.
Wood signifies processes conducive to growth, fruition and decay.
Water signifies, among other things, fructifying functions.

Fire signifies strongly dynamic activities.
Earth signifies supportive, womb-like functions.

All of them are positive and supportive in some circumstances, negative and destructive in others, according to nature's needs.

Every Taoist yogic manual is full of matter dealing with *wu hsing*. A Chinese might be astonished to come upon a book such as this one and find references to *wu hsing* so few. The problem is that their symbolism is so inextricably related to different Chinese ideograms (or parts of ideograms) and to two systems of reckoning known respectively as the Ten Celestial Stems and Twelve Branches that it is difficult indeed to make sense in the English language of the passages concerning them. They have been mentioned here in passing chiefly because people in the West with an interest in Taoism are almost certain to come upon them in relation to some of the sciences related to Taoism, such as *t'ai chi* callisthenics, I Ching divination and Chinese medicine, all of which are now much more widespread in America and Europe than Taoism itself.

(e) THE THREE TREASURES

Taoist yogic manuals have also a great deal to say about what are known as the Three Treasures. These in their coarse form comprise semen, breath and spirit, each of which is held to have a subtle cosmic counterpart. It is by the generation, nourishment and interaction of these six that remarkable yogic powers are attained and preparation made for the ultimate experience, Return to the Source. The practices pertaining to them, known as the Internal Alchemy, unfortunately require the instruction and supervision of a competent teacher; to perform them on one's own would be dangerous to health and would even induce insanity, for which reason the section on Taoist practice in this book deals with them only briefly. However, not every Taoist master considers the Inner Alchemy essential to mystical experience, so perhaps the loss is not as great as it might otherwise be.

(f) GOALS ATTAINABLE BY MIDDLE-LEVEL ADEPTS

Attainment of the ultimate goal, Return to the Source, is so difficult that many Taoist adepts in China were quite content to aim at lesser goals, of a kind that everyone may hope to achieve by diligent cultivation of the Way. If the exercises set forth in this book are not in themselves sufficient to carry one that far, at least they will lead to making some progress in the right direction. The goals naturally include one that is aimed at by almost all serious meditators, namely the attainment of increasingly profound intuitive insights into the nature of reality – insights that are often accompanied by sensations of bliss and invariably result in a deepening of wisdom, of joy in life and greater understanding of life's meaning. Other goals, perhaps to be regarded as incidental to this one, are the prolongation or restoration of youthful vigour, excellent health, and longevity extending to upwards of a hundred years of age that is attended by good health and happiness to the very end.

Longevity in itself might not seem altogether desirable but, in this case, it is likely to go together not only with radiant health but also with a joyous tranquillity that will make every moment of life worth living by banishing the negative reactions commonly aroused by boredom, frustration, bereavement, loss, anxiety and fear. Incidentally, a person who is freed from these reactions is likely to be loved and esteemed, if only because he has no sorrows to inflict upon others who feel they have enough of their own sorrows to bear. Besides, he is sure to develop into a merry person, free from envy and dislike, and therefore much sought after as a friend.

I have no doubt that all of these objectives are well within the bounds of possibility. In many a remote hermitage rising from the slopes of one or other of China's innumerable sacred mountains, I used to come upon Taoist recluses extraordinarily merry, healthy and active for their years, able to perform surprising feats of athletic prowess and often skilled as well in such arts as healing, calligraphy, poetic composition, music, painting, defensive combat or miniature landscape gardening. There was a peacefulness and joyousness about them; merely to be with them for a few days restored one's faith in life's value and opened up new possibilities of happiness. All of these proceeded from a wisdom that comes from inner stillness.

(g) IMMORTALITY AND RETURN TO THE SOURCE

Though we are concerned in this book mainly with the early stages of the Way, these should be understood in relation to the ultimate aims of Taoist yogins. This brings us to their concept of life after death. As a result of interactions between Taoism and Buddhism extending over two millennia, I used to encounter many Taoists who believed that beings undergo a long succession of lives before attaining to full self-realisation; but the more typically Taoist view is quite otherwise. According to early tradition, a man is born with two souls which separate at death, one rising to a celestial region where after a while it disintegrates – though its existence can be greatly prolonged in certain cases – the other sinking into the earth and gradually disintegrating likewise. Therefore, Taoist yogins were impelled by a feeling of urgency to seek the attainment of full self-realisation in this very life as the only sure means of achieving whichever of two high ends they personally believed in.

One of these ends, though termed immortality, actually connotes no more than prolonged existence as an individual in a kind of spiritualised mortal shape, whether in a spiritual realm or in one of the mysterious, inaccessible parts of the earth where immortals are believed to dwell. Delightful though this may be, to desire this state of being is to reveal ignorance of the true nature of the glorious apotheosis known as Return to the Source; for, when that is understood, the joys of relative immortality – however poetic – pale beside it. Those Taoist mystics who, during their contemplative yoga, have already attained to blissful intuitions of the splendour of the highest goal are fortunate indeed; for they are confident of achieving, either at the moment of death or before that, a goal so high that it transcends all the other goals conceived by man since the beginning of history – at least, that is how it seems to me. This grand apotheosis is of so strange a nature that it cannot be conveyed in a sentence, but has to be led up to gradually. To begin with an unsatisfactory and rather primitive analogy, let us say provisionally that the experience must be something like what a raindrop would feel if it were conscious at the actual moment of merging with the ocean; in other words, the adept, suddenly freed from the last shred of the delusion that he has an individual existence of his own, suddenly becomes conscious of his perfect unity with the whole. However, whereas a raindrop falling into the ocean and merging with it indivisibly can never be more than an insignificant part of the infinitude of water all around him, that is by no means parallel to the case of an illumined adept. In the first place, he has never really been apart from the 'ocean' of the Tao; therefore he does not suddenly achieve a new state of union with it, as does the raindrop, but becomes blissfully aware of having never been divided from it. In the second place – and it is this which makes the experience splendid beyond all power of conception – he does not feel himself to be a minute part of the vast ocean but, as it were, *becomes the whole!* It is as though his consciousness suddenly expands beyond its former puny limits *to contain the whole cosmos within itself!* The Tao, being similar in nature not to a vast material body like the ocean's, but rather to something closely resembling mind or pure consciousness, does not have parts to it; the Tao is *wholly present* in each of its smallest fragments; therefore, to become conscious of perfect union with it is to become conscious of actually *being* the entire cosmos, of being in all ways infinite! A man who undergoes this glorious experience must feel as though his consciousness, once seemingly contained within his little skull, has all of a sudden expanded to become coterminous with the whole of existence!

This truth was once conveyed to me by an old gentleman called Tsêng Lao-wêng who as he was speaking looked into my eyes, and for a fraction of a second I seemed to grasp the purport intuitively; in other words, for that brief moment, I actually experienced to some degree how it feels *to be the universe!* But of course I was not ready for so exalted an experience and hurriedly dropped my eyes, feeling that otherwise I should instantly be burnt up by a current so powerful that not even ashes would remain of me. Naturally I had no time then to reflect on the matter in those terms – I am just trying to convey something of the nature of my feeling during that instant, a mixture of bliss and terror. Yet, had I been far advanced along the Way and properly prepared for the experience, then there would have been no terror – only unadulterated bliss. Such then is the meaning of Return to the Source, insofar as mere words can convey a reality lying far beyond the limits of conceptual thought.

3

Attitude

To succeed in yogic practice, one must of course cultivate a proper attitude to people, affairs and the whole environment. A Taoist adept is one who comes to resemble the Three Friends of Winter. Like the pine-tree, he may hope to achieve remarkable longevity. Like the winter-plum-tree, crimson petals gleaming against the snow, he blossoms in adversity, serenely unaffected by chill and drear surroundings. Like the bamboo, he is so strong and yet so flexible that he bends effortlessly to accommodate the prevailing winds of circumstance and, far from being broken by them, springs back again with matchless resilience. Of these three qualities, the last is of paramount importance; it is at this that he must aim, then the others will come of themselves.

To be tense, rigid, uptight, inflexible, unaccommodating, rigorous in conduct and belief, bigoted, humourless, quick to take offence, easily put out, cast down, care-furrowed, complaining, overwhelmed by adversity – all of these are the very antithesis of Taoist qualities. People who pride themselves on being able to swim against the current, to carve against the grain of things, will never make good Taoists, unless they change their attitude. A Taoist conserves his energy by easily according with and adapting himself to each situation. His will may be as strong as the current in a mountain stream, but it does not lead him to press forward uselessly against obstacles that are insuperable or else can be easily circumvented. Caring nothing at all for what people may think of him, he takes no pride in heroism for its own sake, so he looks for the easiest way round. That is not to say that he willingly surrenders an objective, only that he will not attempt the impossible, nor expend more energy than is strictly necessary to attain the possible. By no means lazy, he conserves his powers in order to make the most of them.

A Taoist has no desire for prominence or popular esteem. Though happy to be of service when called upon, he will do what must be done with the minimum of fuss and retire from public notice at the earliest possible moment, well content to let others enjoy the credit. He is the eternal wanderer who tranquilly takes things as they come, putting forth energy when need be, but inwardly relaxed. When things go well, he enjoys them to the full, though rather in the manner of someone charmed by an unexpected vista of primroses in a wood, who rejoices in their fresh beauty for a little while, without the least desire to cling or to possess, and then passes on. When ills befall, he accepts them without repining, knowing very well there can be no up without down, no summer without winter, no growth without decay; besides, he is quick to discover beauty in the seemingly dreary and to find compensations in what to others might appear to be unmitigated ills – rather like a friend of mine who, struck down in middle age by polio, reacted to the doctor's prediction that he would be bedridden all his life by exclaiming: 'Ha, at last I shall have as much time as I want for reading!'

For these and other reasons, there is a special affinity between Taoists and flowing water, which is at once the weakest and the strongest of the elements. Streams are persistent in making for their goal, but do not batter away at obstacles they can circumvent; and, when no way can be found round a wall of rock, they erode it with such patience that the progress of their conquest is often impossible to discern. Where streams running from high ground to low can gush effortlessly, they gush; on level ground, where they have become broad and wide, their motion is often invisible, yet never falters. I believe Lao-tzû had water in mind when he wrote: 'The weakest thing in heaven and earth strikes against and overcomes the strongest. Coming from nowhere [i.e. invisibly in the form of vapour], it penetrates where there is no crack [i.e. through minute pores in the rock]. Thus do I know the value of *wu wei* [literally, 'no activity']. The teaching without words and the value of *wu wei* are not often recognised by the world.'

Wu wei, a favourite Taoist term, is difficult to translate satisfactorily and has led to many misunderstandings about the proper method of cultivating the Way. I think it means no activity that is not rooted in the nature of a situation, no wasteful exertion. Nature, who was Lao-tzû's beloved teacher, is perpetually involved in activity, but not of an unnecessary kind. Trees growing in the shade bend towards the sunlight; all plants draw nourishment from earth and sky; birds build nests and hunt worms to feed themselves and their young; squirrels store nuts for use in winter; fish swim and tigers leap – but these are actions in response to need, to the exigencies of Here and Now. They do not proceed from calculation or from a desire for pre-eminence, power, pelf or profit, nor are they carried to excess. A deer can stand grazing safely under the eyes of a tiger, if the tiger has had a meal to satisfy him. True, certain fish are said to lay eggs by the million, but that prodigality is in response to an actual need in parts of the ocean where an egg's chances of survival are very close to nil. None of these activities contravenes the principle of *wu wei*, whereas cornering a market or seeking to be one up on someone does not accord with it.

A Taoist's needs are few and simple. Food can be nourishing and tasty without the addition of exotic or unusually expensive ingredients; garments can suit the climate and be attractive without being unduly numerous or made of costly fabrics; one can get along very comfortably without platinum or diamonds, which in any case are tiresome because they need to be guarded so carefully; and one can make a room or dwelling quite charming without going to great expense. In short, there is no advantage – but there are several serious disadvantages – in having too much of anything, and in acquiring and looking after rare and costly possessions. Followers of the Way know instinctively how to combine enjoyment of modest comfort and beauty with a taste for frugality; above all, they shun ostentation.

I have to admit that, though Taoism offers an admirable way of life for the individual, it does not have specific means of solving the mass problems that afflict our great cities; these require mass remedies beyond an individual's power to provide. Even so, just as a murky puddle is made a trifle less opaque by every drop of pure rain or dew that falls there, so is the quality of dense urban communities improved by every individual who stays unblemished by greed, acquisitiveness, extravagance, envy and crooked dealing. If ever Taoist values come to be cherished by large numbers of individuals in the West, especially if some of them are people in positions of power, society as a whole as well as those individuals will benefit.

The relaxed, good-humoured tolerance that characterises followers of the Way makes them loath to be interfering. Quietly pursuing their goals, happy to share their wisdom with anyone who comes of his own accord to ask for help or advice, they are content to leave others entirely free to live their lives as seems best to them, to 'do their own thing'. Taoist masters are reluctant to put themselves forward in the capacity of missionaries or busybodies; indeed, they are so apt to shun the limelight that their next-door neighbours may remain quite unaware of living in the vicinity of a sage. This is undoubtedly one of the reasons why they are so hard to find. A Chinese friend of mine with considerable influence in Taoist and Buddhist circles recently failed to persuade some learned followers of the Way in Taiwan to visit

America, where plenty of people would have felt honoured and delighted to look after them. Under present circumstances, this total lack of missionary spirit is rather unfortunate, but Western followers of the Way would do well to hide their light under a bushel; eagerness to be proclaimed a guru has no place in a Taoistic attitude to life. As Lao-tzû said of the sages of old, 'They were retiring and hesitant as though shy of the people all around them, and they treated everybody with respect as one treats an honoured guest.' To this day, one does not find a true Taoist sage proclaiming 'I know all about the Tao. If you want to attain the goal, you had better enrol among my students.' Self-advertisement is so foreign to the Taoist spirit that it is really hard to find a teacher, but that is better than having a lot of self-proclaimed teachers who, having little real knowledge, are likely to lead enthusiastic students astray. Moreover, it provides a criterion for judging what teachers *not* to follow, namely anyone who makes extravagant claims to be far advanced along the Way. On the other hand, if some good teachers do arrive and let their lineage be known, that is another matter, for that kind of information can generally be checked. By lineage is meant the names of the teacher's own teacher, his teacher's teacher and so on back for perhaps many generations. In China, discovering a teacher's spiritual lineage was one of the ways of ascertaining that he had something worth while to teach. In course of time, there may well be Westerners qualified to teach much more advanced yogas than those contained in this book, and one of the ways of recognising them initially will be to discover the names of the teachers who instructed them.

B   PRACTICE

1

Mode of Living and Preparations

(a) GENERAL

The earliest Taoists known to history were wanderers in a literal sense; their spiritual descendants still like to describe themselves as wandering through life, though this has long since become a euphemism meaning just that they take life as it comes, welcoming its ups, tranquilly accepting its downs as an inevitable part of the grand whole, clinging to nothing whatsoever. Some two millennia ago, those early wanderers were succeeded by communities of recluses who built their hermitages in remote spots notable for scenic beauty, so as to have seclusion and ideal surroundings for cultivating the Way. Others lived as ordinary householders observing their family obligations and earning their living variously like other people. There have never been stringent rules restricting modes of living. Taoists do not care for restrictions; besides, so much of their practice relates to cultivating an attitude of mind and achieving inner stillness that surroundings are of secondary importance, except that living amidst scenes of natural beauty remote from the bustle and din of cities does make practice much easier. Under present-day conditions, there is seldom much choice; most people have to live in places that fit the circumstances of their lives.

(b) DIET

The chief dietary rule for Taoist adepts (as for serious meditators of all kinds) is to eat abstemiously. The Taoist communities I visited in China ate well if they could afford to, but always lightly. In the south, rice was their staple food; in the north, this was replaced by wheat or other grains taken in the form of porridge, bread and noodles. The

dishes that accompanied these basic foods consisted mostly of vegetables, cooked with beancurd and a little meat, poultry or fish and
flavoured with products gathered locally in the mountains – mush-
rooms, bamboo shoots, tree-ears (a delicious kind of fungus), herbs,
water-chestnuts, berries, nuts and fruit. No foods were specially
prohibited but, since many of the recluses were learned in Chinese
traditional medicine, they knew which foods are nourishing and
which are best avoided or taken only sparingly. Nothing in their
philosophy discouraged them from enjoying tasty dishes and drinking
a little wine or spirit at meal-times; however, as the aims of their yogic
regime included living to a great age while sustaining unblemished
health and comparatively youthful vigour, they took care to avoid
excess in eating and drinking, as in everything else, and to ensure that
their rather light diet was nourishing. Costly foods or those brought
with difficulty from far-off places were on the whole eschewed.

   Western adepts would do well to eat simply and avoid heavy meals,
but not to set their faces puritanically against tasty cooking. Rigid
asceticism and overindulgence are both departures from the Way; so,
too, is over-concern about what to eat and not eat such as one
commonly finds in California these days, for concern leads to anxiety,
which is as harmful to physical and mental health as a slow poison.
Taoism inculcates a relaxed attitude to just about everything.

(c) INTOXICANTS

Taoist adepts, though they drink wine and spirits in moderation
especially when the weather is damp or cold, regard even occasional
drunkenness as a departure from the Way, since it is not good for
health and far from conducive to progress in yogic meditation.
Moreover, alcohol is never taken except as an accompaniment to
eating; they would not be tempted by cocktails before dinner, or by
spirits taken after dinner and before going to bed. That tobacco is not
listed as a harmful substance in the yogic manuals is due to the fact
that they were written long before tobacco smoking became prevalent
in China. Tobacco *is* harmful yogically, because not conducive to the
best functioning of the respiratory system; breath is one of the yogin's
Three Treasures, which have to be guarded, nourished, refined and
kept from all polluting influences as far as possible. As to hashish,
'hard' and psychedelic drugs, these are not regarded as a legitimate
way of attaining to higher states of consciousness. There is no
denying that they do sometimes have that effect, but their action is

difficult to control, their effects on the psychic channels are harmful, and the exalted states of consciousness they sometimes give rise to are of no help in attaining the permanent expansion of consciousness at which yogins aim. It would be hard indeed to find a meditator well on the way to self-realisation who would sanction the use of such drugs by people who hope to progress far along the Way. It has been amply demonstrated that there are no short cuts to high yogic attainment. (Where certain drugs do have a limited usefulness is in convincing newcomers to the Way that there *are* higher states of consciousness to be attained, but their action is too uncertain for one to count upon them to do even this much.)

(d) SEX

Few Taoists take vows of chastity. Taoist recluses are not monks, although a fair number of them choose to practice celibacy, especially upon the higher stages of the path, because the energies of body and mind are so closely interlinked that prodigal expenditure of one form of energy reduces the total store available for use in yogic cultivation. On the other hand, it would not occur to a Taoist to equate sexual intercourse with sin, it being a natural function. It is realised that rigid abstention can be harmful to people as yet so far from a high level of spiritual attainment as to find absolute celibacy disturbing to their meditations. Suppressed longings and tortured fantasies can undermine mental and physical health to a much greater extent than carefully regulated sexual indulgence, which is therefore held to be consonant with cultivation of the Way, especially during the early stages of progress.

The accent is on moderation, because frequent seminal emission so depletes one's store of one of the Three Treasures as to negate the benefits of yogic practice. To avoid the harm that may in some circumstances be caused by strict chastity on the one hand, and to inhibit overfrequent seminal emission on the other, Taoists advocate a regime of continence. This term, which has a very particular Taoist connotation, implies no limits to frequency of sexual intercourse as such; what is meant is that intercourse should be made to stop short of seminal emission, except at comparatively rare intervals that increase in length with each decade starting from the age of puberty. Curiously, the teaching that physical and mental energy are depleted by incontinent intercourse does not apply to women; the passage in the *Tao Tê Ching* asserting that 'the valley spirit is inexhaustible' is taken to mean, among many other things, that a woman's essence (which, in its coarse form, is sexual energy) is incapable of depletion because of its power of self-renewal.

The sexual yogas advocated by the followers of some schools of Taoism involve very strict male continence. Belonging to the category of advanced yogas, they are never practised without the instruction of a qualified teacher; and, as there are many other schools of Taoist thought that deem this type of yoga to be useless or positively harmful to progress along the Way, I have thought it best not to present them, even in a simplified form.

(e) MIND AND BODY

All that was taught in the section on Taoist attitude should be thoroughly mastered at the outset and worked upon until a right attitude becomes instinctive. Unless one becomes relaxed, flexible, fond of simplicity and frugality, reverent towards nature and towards everyone and everything in the whole cosmic environment, the Way remains blocked. Failure to acquire such an attitude ranks with continuing rigidity of any kind, and with inability to overcome anxiety, as an indication that there is something wrong with one's practice, that progress has been halted or disquietingly slowed down. Effective yoga is, above all, directed at attaining exalted states of mind; and, since matter is but one of mind's manifestations, all that pertains to the body is of secondary importance. Physical health and longevity are sought by Taoists not for their own sake, but because the former is necessary to mental health and emotional equilibrium, while living to a vigorous old age allows the adept more time in which to attain to full self-realisation – a goal that relates to a state of mind, not of body.

Nevertheless, the claims to attention of the body must by no means be disregarded. Its health is nourished by abstemiousness in eating, drinking and sexual intercourse, by correct breathing, appropriate exercise, adequate cleanliness and avoidance of every kind of excess. There are Taoist physical exercises that produce quite extraordinary results, causing adepts to become unbelievably hardy and vigorous for their age and to retain a remarkably youthful appearance. As masters qualified to give instruction in this matter seem not yet to have appeared in the West, it will be best for adepts to practise *t'ai chi*, for teachers are comparatively easy to find in both America and Europe and this type of exercise, being firmly based on Taoist principles, is capable of producing all the results just mentioned, besides being suitable to embark upon at any age. For example, the skills of my 'Chinese nephew', Huang Chung-liang (Al Huang), stop only a little short of flying and he has maintained the physique of a man twenty years younger than his age. His mother, a *t'ai chi* master of the Pa Kua School, is still a youthful person, although already in her sixties. Conversely, exercises of the Swedish drill or sergeant-major type must at all costs be avoided by an adept, as these induce strain, which is the very opposite of what is required by followers of the Way. *T'ai chi* was evolved by recluses famous for extraordinary feats; and it is based on the concepts of maintaining a proper balance among the Three Powers (heaven, earth and man) and the Five Activities symbolised my metal, wood, water, fire and earth. Nothing could be more typically Taoist than *t'ai chi* and yet it is thoroughly up to date, as Master Huang's adaptations of *t'ai chi* to ballet clearly illustrate. *Judo*, *kendo* and *taekwando*, all evolved from the same principles as *t'ai chi*, are also acceptable substitutes for Taoist physical training, provided that a spirit of fierce competitiveness and desire to win does not supplant the Taoist ideal of taking the rough with the smooth. The idea is not to win, but merely to do the best one can and then abide tranquilly by the result of a contest. Disturbance of spirit is inimical to progress along the Way.

The special instructions for bathing contained in some Taoist manuals advocate using certain hours of the day, days of the month, etc., and certain rhythms in the act of pouring water over oneself; all these relate to the Taoist science of numbers which many advanced adepts regard as having no real importance. The main points to bear in mind are that health requires cleanliness and that bathing, as a preparation for mind-cleansing meditation, has a powerful supportive effect.

Lastly, it is laid down that the adept should at all times dress suitably for the weather; avoid unnecessary exposure to extremes of heat, cold and wet; and be careful not to sleep too much or too little, or at widely fluctuating times. In short, he should take common sense as a guide to the nourishing, development, cleansing and resting of his physical frame which, being interlinked with his mind to an extent seldom recognised by spiritual teachers schooled in Western traditions, may be rightly considered to be an extension of it.

(f) SURROUNDINGS

Taoist recluses were apt to spend a lot of time out of doors communing with nature; in good weather, they generally preferred to perform their yogic meditation practice in the open air, deeming this to be favourable to circulation of the *ch'i*. Beautiful scenery – rocks, trees, flowers, streams, waterfalls and mountains – induces tranquillity of mind. However, in bad weather or under urban conditions, cultivation of the Way can proceed very well indoors. As ritual and actual purity are very important, the early hours of the morning when the *ch'i* circulates without impediment are deemed ideal for practice; so adepts generally begin the day by rising very early, evacuating their bowels, cleansing their mouths and bathing, during which they avoid distracting thoughts and states of mind likely to hinder meditation, which becomes increasingly easy to do as progress along the Way progresses.

A place intended for regular yogic use should be kept both ritually and physically pure; that is to say no polluting influences should be allowed to enter, and the place itself, together with any objects it contains, should be kept scrupulously clean. Therefore, a special room (or special corner of a room) should be reserved exclusively for yogic practice, so that an atmosphere of physical and ritual purity can be strictly maintained. In a dwelling of more than one storey, this room or corner should be on the highest floor; but, in a one-floor apartment, all that is necessary is to choose a place to which guests are not likely to penetrate, so that its purity can be maintained without the embarrassment of having to call their attention to its sacred function. Sacred things should not be allowed to excite derision; if the adept should happen to cause this by drawing special attention to them, the responsibility will be his alone. Therefore his practice and everything pertaining to it should be as unostentatious as possible. One cannot tell people not to smoke or think certain thoughts in a particular place, or not to use an incense-burner as an ashtray, without the risk of exciting derision. To be a Taoist adept is to be much like an iceberg, not at all in the sense of being cold, but of keeping a great deal hidden from the gaze of ordinary people. Ordinary people, as manifestations of the Tao, are by no means to be despised, but one does not reveal to them matters they are as yet not ready to understand and respect.

No special adjuncts are needed in the meditation room (or corner), but a few symbolical objects to mark its apartness from other places are deemed helpful. Though it should be plain and uncluttered, one may like to have a vase of tastefully arranged flowers or branches covered with fruit blossom, or a dwarf tree or miniature rockery in an earthenware container, or perhaps a picture or a scroll. For this last, suitable subjects include a beautiful landscape, a gathering of Taoist immortals, a painted *yin–yang* symbol, or the Chinese character for

Tao brushed in fine calligraphy, or a striking passage from the *Tao Tê Ching*. It is usual to start each meditation period by lighting a stick of incense and planting it upright in a bronze or porcelain incense-burner tightly packed with ash – an ordinary bowl will do. The incense should not have a very sweet or strongly pungent perfume, but smell like very fragrant wood rather than, say, roses or lilies. One can do well without any incense at all, but it provides a link with a very ancient tradition and has more than symbolic significance. Symbolically the thin wavering plume of smoke represents the soaring of spiritual aspiration and evokes the idea of energy being released from matter to infuse the upper air; in addition, it is somehow helpful in inducing a meditative state of mind, which is doubtless why the ancients made use of it in this way. Adjuncts of this kind are not despised by those who understand their purpose and significance. Though certain passages in Zen works have caused a good many Westerners to suppose that ritual is rather a hindrance than a help to spiritual progress, it is noteworthy that not a single temple in Japan or anywhere throughout Buddhist Asia dispenses with ritual altogether. It is certainly a hindrance to understanding if one supposes that a ritual practice properly performed can *of itself* be spiritually effective, but not if one takes such practices as aids to inducing a desired state of mind, for then their efficacy is very similar to that of works of art which have ennobling effects on those who contemplate them.

2

Basic Meditative Techniques

(a) PURPOSES

The instructions regarding sitting are to be observed in all the meditations given in part I of this book when they are practised in a formal manner. However, some of the practices can also be performed informally with very great benefit; in that case, any posture will serve, for one can meditate whether walking, standing, sitting or lying. Indeed, contemplation of nature is a yogic exercise that can perhaps be best approached informally. There is never any need to make a fetish of the sitting posture; I do not go along with those teachers who claim that the leg pains resulting from sitting in the lotus posture are an aid to effective meditation. The Taoist emphasis on being always relaxed and avoiding strain extends no less to contemplative yoga than to any other activity. On the other hand, if one can comfortably maintain the lotus posture (sitting with legs crossed, soles of the feet facing upwards like those of a Buddha statue), so much the better, as it is held to be the position most conducive to long and successful sitting for those who can maintain it without being racked with pain; besides making it less likely that the meditator will fall asleep, it can be maintained by experts for days at a time (should that ever be necessary), and it assists the circulation of *ch'i* throughout the body, as well as inducing stillness of mind. The purpose of informal meditation, which does not involve special sitting and breathing techniques, is to enable the adept to make good use of all those odd intervals throughout the day when he happens to be unoccupied, and to combine his practice with strolling about to enjoy the beauties of nature. This method also makes it possible to meditate anywhere one may chance to be without calling unwelcome attention to oneself. Though Taoists are very odd people by worldly standards, they prefer to pass by unnoticed.

(b) SITTING

Few Taoist masters are very strict about meditation posture. The lotus posture is ideal, if it can be maintained without discomfort. Sitting in half-lotus (with the sole of only one foot facing upwards) or simply with the legs crossed tailor-fashion is also acceptable. All these positions are easier to maintain painlessly over considerable lengths of time if one places upon a large square meditation cushion a smaller cushion to raise the buttocks and thus reduce pressure on the legs. As the bodies of Western people differ from those of Asians, especially as regards bone structure, it may be advisable for this second and smaller cushion to be much higher than the low flat kind traditionally used (see illustration on p. 160). In America I observed that many Western meditators were able to maintain their postures comfortably by this means. Elderly beginners and physically handicapped people may prefer to use a chair. In that case, the height should be such that the upper part of the adept's legs is parallel to the floor. The ankles and knees should be lightly touching to ensure the free circulation of *ch'i*. The hands should rest on the lap in one of the two positions given below. From the hips upward, the position of the body is the same as for meditators sitting cross-legged and, unless a physical handicap makes it absolutely necessary, one should not make use of the arms and back of the chair. Therefore a wooden stool of the right height, covered by a thin flat cushion, is probably best.

Circulation of *ch'i* is best ensured by having the hands rest lightly on the lap and in contact with each other. Either the back of the right hand should be cupped in the palm of the left hand with the tips of the thumbs and forefingers of each hand joined to form adjacent circles; or else the fists, lightly clenched with the knuckles facing outward, should rest side by side, right thumb extended and embraced by the fingers of the left hand. The body should be held straight, but certainly not rigidly, with the head bent *very slightly* forward, eyes three-quarters closed, mouth shut, upper and lower teeth not quite touching, tip of the tongue in contact with the centre of the upper gum. The posture should be entirely free from tension, yet not so relaxed as to encourage drowsiness.

Traditionally, a long loose robe worn over soft baggy trousers was the normal garb for meditation, but all that really matters is that one's clothes should be loose and comfortable. Belts, collars, etc., should on no account be tight, nor body and legs exposed to currents of cold air. If a robe long enough to cover the legs completely is not worn, a light rug may be placed over the legs in winter as a protection against draughts.

(c) BREATHING

Of the characteristic Taoist yogic breathing exercises, most cannot be usefully or safely practised without a teacher, but there are some from which everyone can derive benefit without the least danger. It is good to commence every yogic meditation with the following exercise, which helps to establish stillness of mind and to promote the circulation of *ch'i*. Like most kinds of yogic breathing, it is also beneficial when practised on its own for ten or fifteen minutes at a time, several times a day, but especially in the early morning.

The adept, having taken up his meditation posture and allowed himself time to feel relaxed in it, starts by taking a series of comparatively deep breaths, somewhat more prolonged than his normal breathing, yet not extremely slow. The time taken for inhalation and exhalation should be exactly the same, and there should be no perceptible pause between them. Respiration should become so regular and calm that the hairs in the nostrils are hardly disturbed; also it should be inaudible even to the breather. This type of breathing should be continued for a few minutes without change, with the attention concentrated wholly upon the passage of air (and *ch'i*) through the outer gateway of the nostrils. If meditation is to follow, the adept presently allows the pace of respiration to return to normal rather gradually, but making sure that (i) his breathing does not become too shallow; (ii) inhalation and exhalation are evenly balanced; and (iii) the process remains quite inaudible. Having attended to this, he should not mar his meditation by further anxiety about his manner of breathing.

If breathing yoga is being performed not as a prelude to meditation, but for its own sake, the adept – once he has thoroughly mastered the method just set forth – may vary it by holding his breath for a while between inhalation and exhalation, though not for longer than it takes him to count rather slowly up to five, for longer pauses are dangerous without the supervision of a teacher. When this second technique has been practised over a period of several weeks, he may experiment cautiously with a breathing practice that is uniquely Taoist. That is to say, he should breathe in and out rather slowly and deeply as in the first practice, meanwhile drawing his stomach well *in* during *inhalation* and pushing it *out* during *exhalation* – the exact opposite of the instinctive order. Acquiring this special technique will stand him in good stead if, later on, he has the good fortune to receive instruction from a teacher qualified to supervise and develop this special type of yogic breathing.

The aim of commencing each meditation session with a few minutes of breathing practice is, first, to calm the mind and stimulate the flow of *ch'i* by concentrating one's whole awareness upon the inflow and outflow of breath; second, to insure that the meditator breathes correctly throughout the session, as very great advantage results from this. Stillness of mind and a rhythmic flow of *ch'i* are hardly possible for as long as breathing remains too shallow or erratic; besides, correct breathing gradually becomes part of the adept's second nature, whereafter it is superfluous to allot several minutes of a session to breath control.

Success in yogic practice and the enjoyment of outstandingly good health both demand attention to breathing which, at all times of the day and night, should be regular, silent and rather deep than shallow. The tendency for people engaged in sedentary occupations to respire only with the upper part of their lungs should be corrected. In course of time, the adept will have become so accustomed to correct breathing as to be able to take relatively arduous exercise without much disturbance to its rhythm. I have known Taoist swordsmen to emerge from a strenuous armed bout, during which bodies and limbs moved seemingly at lightning speed, with their breathing so far from laboured that they might have just awakened from a refreshing sleep.

(d) STILLNESS OF MIND

Stilling the mind is the method, and stillness the goal, of many kinds of contemplative practice. Seldom is stillness easy to achieve. One may close the doors of the senses, as Chuang-tzû advises, by withdrawing awareness from one's surroundings and causing the waves of thought to subside; but consciousness cannot be totally without an object, or it ceases to be consciousness. Yet teachers of yoga do speak often of objectless awareness. What they mean by this term is best illustrated by comparing the meditator's awareness to a lantern casting its rays on a limitless expanse of pure white snow. The lantern's brightness is not dimmed, that is to say that the adept remains keenly alert; but its rays are diffused over undifferentiated purity, that is, the object of awareness is the entire field of being, not one or more of its differentiated forms. Into a mind thus fixed upon the hidden aspect of the Tao drops little by little, yet with gathering momentum, the intuitive wisdom that leads ultimately to what Taoists call Return to the Source and Buddhists, Enlightenment. In

Taoist terms, the child communicates directly with the mother and is, for a while, absorbed in her.

It may prove difficult to reach this state, so all kinds of techniques have been devised, such as concentrating awareness on the rhythm of the breathing or the pulsing of blood, or else on one of the body's psychic centres, especially the Dark Gate lying just behind the mid-point between the eyes, or the centre located in the middle of the body on a level with the navel. All of these promote total concentration on a single sensation or object in the expectation that it will ultimately dissolve into formlessness, and infinity be grasped. Moreover, for an adept still at the early stages of the Way, merely to retain one-pointed concentration for a little while is excellent in itself.

Another method of approach is to think of oneself as an empty vessel waiting to be filled. One visualises the Tao, in this context, as an infinite ocean of being-non-being which will pour into a vessel as soon as impediments to its flow have been removed. One reflects: 'Here am I about to enter a state of pure emptiness with my whole being opened up to the splendour that will presently fill me'; but if, after a while, one sees flashing lights or experiences a sensation of flying, this must not be allowed to lead to a state of pride in accomplishment, for that would inevitably drag the mind down into the depths of egoism and delusion. After all, what happens is not due to the adept's puny powers, but to the illimitable Tao, of which the adept himself is no more than a fleeting manifestation. At all times 'self' must maintain a very low profile, for 'self' is not really a person called Smith or Huang, but the self of the sublime Tao of which Smith and Huang are transient manifestations. Pride in temporary success is a great enemy of yogic progress and leads to rapid downfall. Remain impervious to such petty feelings. Just be still!

(e) TIME

Newcomers to yoga should not strain themselves by overexertion. Twenty minutes or so in the early morning and again in the evening is sufficient for a start, provided that practice is absolutely regular. Gradually the time of each session and the number of sessions can be increased until, at an advanced stage, it is nothing extraordinary to find oneself meditating for a day or two at a time without a break. This will develop of itself. There is no need to force the pace. Eagerness to succeed is self-defeating. Absolute regularity of practice is worth far more than occasional lengthy sessions. The Tao is rhythmical in its workings, so too the well instructed adept. (Informal meditation can, of course, be performed at any time as often as one wishes, whether wandering through a forest or lying sleepless in bed, but it should not take the place of the regular daily sessions.)

(f) A STORY

Once a brilliant young scholar surnamed Li left home on a sudden impulse to become the pupil of a famous master. Welcoming him in some surprise to his mountain retreat, the master inquired: 'Young Sir, what has this poor old fellow got to teach a learned gentleman like you?' Hurriedly prostrating himself at the master's feet, Li cried: 'I have studied the Four Books and Five Classics (of State Confucianism) from end to end without discovering a single thing that could set me on the road to immortality.'

'And just why should you wish to become an immortal?' retorted the master. 'I have never heard of immortals being accorded high rank in the government of the Empire, whereas a Confucian scholar of your calibre might end up as a Minister of State.' Nevertheless, the young man's obvious sincerity won the day and the master consented to teach him.

Within a few months, Li had become proficient in yogic practices and thought nothing of rising from his body to visit the cloud palaces of the immortals or to wing his way '*hsi-hsi* through the air' and circle round the sun and moon. 'I believe I am well on the way to outdistancing the master,' he reflected. 'Already I am close to being an immortal. Ah, the bliss of knowing how to fly without wings!'

Emboldened by this thought, he suggested to the master that they should have a race. 'Without rising from his meditation mat, each of us shall fly to the abode of immortals on Kun Lung Mountain [far away in central Asia], pluck one of the peaches of longevity and return as fast as possible. Whoever comes back first with one of those rare fruit shall have the pleasure of entertaining the other to a moonlight feast.'

'Good,' replied the master, smiling. 'Let us go to our cells and begin at once.' Needless to say, the old gentleman had scarcely crossed his legs in meditation than he was away to Kun Lung and back again with a fragrant peach nestling in his hand. Hours later, he went in to see if Li's spirit was still absent from his body, only to find the unfortunate scholar close to tears; for, try as he would, his spirit had stubbornly refused to rise even as far as the ceiling of his cell.

'My power has deserted me,' he cried.

'Not at all,' replied the master. 'It is the power of the Tao that has deserted you, because you ascribed its marvellous functioning to yourself. Now you will have to start again at the very beginning.'

The moral of this allegory is that adepts, however much they welcome the wonderful experiences that sometimes visit them, should not pride themselves on any personal achievement, since only in a very superficial sense could such an achievement be called their own.

3

Intimate Communion with Nature

(a) PURPOSE

To overcome an individual's delusion of apartness through direct intuitive perception of his essential unity with nature's being, to learn to live in harmonious accord with *all* of nature's workings, to free the mind of turgid thoughts and thus achieve the permanent state of inner stillness required for cultivation of the Way.

(b) PREPARATION

True wisdom is essentially a product of the 'wordless teaching' so highly esteemed by Lao-tzû; hence yogic progress has seldom been dependent on book learning, which more often constitutes a hindrance than an aid. Nevertheless, books are needed to indicate the direction to which the mind must turn. I believe that Western students of the Way will find in the writings of Ralph Waldo Emerson a bridge between their own heritage of learning and Lao-tzû's subtle perception of the being of nature and nature of being. They would do well to ponder appropriate sections of the *Tao Tê Ching* (of which there are now many English versions) in conjunction with a study of Emerson's philosophy.

(c) TAKING THE ROUGH WITH THE SMOOTH

Frequent contemplation of the natural environment leads to loving appreciation of nature in all her moods. Cyclones, devastating floods, forest fires, icy deluges of sleet and hail, though often catastrophic, are as necessary to nature's pattern as warm sunshine, spring rain and gentle breezes. Destruction and creation are two sides of the same coin. Dense forests, for example, would perish for lack of breathing space but for the periodic occurrence of forest fires; good soil would lose its capacity to nourish if deprived of the organic matter resulting from the death of plants; and so on. Nature is not concerned with individuals, but with the well-being of the whole. The yearly cycle involves generation, growth, decay and dissolution, with the *yang* principle dominant for half the year, whereafter it gradually succumbs to the onset of *yin*. For Taoists, all seasons have their charm, each being unique but not superior or inferior to the others. Close intimacy with nature leads to our appreciating its ferocity no less than its benignity, and thus to clear insight into the grand pattern of being. Whereas gardeners are dismayed by weeds and travellers by wind and snow, the Taoist adept welcomes all that comes along; plunged deeply into the mystery of being, he sees in every change a miraculous manifestation of the workings of the sublime Tao. As the source and content of all energy, spirit and matter, the very 'stuff of being', the Tao creates and destroys on a vast scale, yet never adding to or subtracting from the whole.

It is good to walk through fields, forests and mountains pondering these matters, eyes wide open to whatever may befall, for this helps to induce a permanent state of mind that has very important consequences for the adept. When he encounters setbacks in his own life or is beset by such seeming ills as sickness, approaching death, loss, bereavement and so on, his serenity remains undisturbed, for to him all manifestations of the Tao are spiritually nourishing. Regret and anxiety have no place in a mind nourished on daily reminders of the simple truth that there can be no smooth without rough, no ups without downs. It is helpful to yogic practice if, during his wanderings through natural settings, the adept takes particular concrete illustrations of this truth as objects of meditation. Having observed this or that phenomenon, he ponders over it for a while, then applies the lesson first to his own circumstances and later, by extension, to a wider field, which he gradually expands to include the entire cosmos. This type of contemplation sometimes leads to experiencing profound intuitions not communicable in words; moreover, a state of bliss may supervene.

(d) PERCEIVING THE ENVIRONMENT AS AN EXTENSION OF ONESELF

Unlike animals, man (especially modern man with his highly

developed self-consciousness) suffers from the delusion of apartness from his environment and from the people it contains. Apartness is a delusion because it implies separation from the Tao, which is impossible. A Taoist method of combating it is as follows. The adept selects some particular manifestation of the eternal Nameless, such as a willow tree, and spends some time each day throughout successive seasons sitting before it rapt in contemplation. He seeks to penetrate its being, to feel his way into its 'willowness', until, as it were, he *becomes* the tree, actually experiencing its sensations such as when the sap is rising or when new green burgeons from its naked branches; its reactions to sunshine, rain or snow; its craving for sustenance from earth and sky and the satisfaction of appeasing hunger. Increasingly as the days go by and the seasons change, the adept will perceive that willow (and, thus, all natural phenomena) to be an extension of his own being, once seemingly bounded by his skin but now not even by the horizon. Meanwhile, his ego-ghost will diminish or slink away, leaving its former victim to blissful enjoyment of the splendour of limitless being.

Even people quite ignorant of yogic cultivation can, if they give their minds to it, perceive depth upon depth of beauty in each season of the year – the reawakening of life in spring, the lushness of summer, the splendours of autumn, the sparkle of early frost followed by the brilliant whiteness of snow piled upon stubble, branches, roofs, and the lovely tracery of naked boughs against the winter sky – but, for the yogin, there are greater joys than all of these. He ceases to be a spectator and becomes part of the scene like those tiny figures perched amidst wastes of rock and mountain one sees in Taoist paintings. Yet he does not feel himself to be an insignificant part of the whole scene, for the whole is mysteriously perceived to be in him, and he in it.

(e) FREEING THE MIND FROM TURGID THOUGHTS AND ATTAINING INNER STILLNESS

Rapt contemplation of nature's beauties and varied aspects leads effortlessly to the calming of turgid thoughts. The mind, rising above man's petty concerns, grows limpid. The leaping waves of thought, as though shamed by nature's immensity, subside. Sounds hitherto scarcely noticed, such as the soughing of wind in the pines, the creak of bamboo, the chirping of tiny insects, the patter of fine raindrops, the lap of running water against rocks and pebbles, will be heard with new ears and seem like soft echoes of the music of the spheres. Into the stillness, drop by drop, will fall intimations of that wisdom beyond mere knowledge that is man's greatest and often most neglected treasure. The adept should sit quietly and so give himself up to the sights and sounds around him that his own being scarcely enters the periphery of his consciousness; the colours of the trees and the gurgling of the stream seem to be there of themselves, to require no co-operation from his senses, of which he is no longer aware. In time, these too may fade away until nothing remains from horizon to horizon and beyond but the white snow of meditation. The essential formlessness of the Tao is now directly apprehended. This is true stillness of mind, the gateway to the wisdom of the teaching without words.

(f) PRACTISING NATURE MYSTICISM

As perceived by Wordsworth, Tennyson, Emerson and other poets and philosophers steeped in nature's secrets, each single flower, each grain of sand contains within itself the whole being of the cosmos. This is a secret one may sometimes stumble upon by oneself, whereat it becomes very obvious and simple, but there is absolutely no way of getting at it through conceptual thought, still less through words. One may know it for a fact through direct experience and roundly assert that it is so, but one can no more explain it to a person lacking that experience than convey a sense of colour to those born blind. The nearest approach to a written explanation of it that has come my way is contained in a book called *The Buddhist Doctrine of Totality*, a work on the *Hua Yen Sutra* by Garma C. C. Chang. Understanding of this secret, except in those rare cases where it dawns unaided, is best achieved through yogic contemplation of a kind that transcends logical thought, though it can sometimes be assisted by wise reflections at the level of conceptual thinking; these – frequently repeated over a varying period of time – may perhaps give rise to a sudden leap of intuition that carries one the rest of the way to full comprehension. Such a prelude to intuition may run more or less as follows. Sitting in meditation posture, one reflects:

'This flower in my hand, though its existence is fleeting, is in a very real sense an actual flower with its own substance, colour, form and smell. Yet these qualities do not belong to it, being dependent on a great variety of factors pertaining to the totality of being, such as the eye and consciousness of a beholder, the quality of light prevailing at the moment, its position relative to my eye and so on. Since any change in one or more of these factors will result in alteration of the flower's colour and/or form, it is clear that those qualities are not inherent in the flower itself. Nor can it be said to have any particular size, being large in relation to some things, small in relation to others, and variable in relation to its distance from my eye. Its one fixed quality would seem to be the nature of its substance, yet even that is illusory as all substances, however much they differ mutually, are in fact manifestations of the non-substance of the Tao, which is intangible, possesses no density and has no differentiated characteristics whatsoever. While I hold this flower in my hand, the Tao is in effect grasping the Tao; while I observe it with my eye and inhale its fragrance with my nose, the Tao is in effect observing and inhaling the Tao. . . .'

Musing along these lines, the adept comes to understand the ultimate emptiness of form, the essential absence of all distinguishing qualities. Next he reflects that the non-substance of the Tao (and therefore of the flower) is, like an ocean of pure consciousness, not subject to limitations of time and space. To speak of the ocean of consciousness as having *parts* to it makes no sense, for one cannot take a knife and cut off a section of mind. The flower, then, cannot be described as an infinitesimal fraction of the non-substance of the Tao; since it shares the Tao's being but cannot be a part of it, it has to *be* the Tao. Beyond this point, conceptual thought must be abandoned; the adept sits in silence, mind stilled, with his awareness wholly concentrated on the flower. The flower is what it is. He no longer tries to reason about it, but just sits peacefully and looks. It would be surprising if, at the first attempt, he were able to take a sudden intuitive leap and penetrate to the heart of the secret then and there; but if he repeats this meditation, preferably at the same time each day over a period of time, he may be visited by brief flashes of intuition and then, one day, suddenly grasp the full meaning of the statement that, just as the cosmos contains the flower, so does the flower contain the cosmos – whereafter, of course, the matter will seem to him quite laughably *simple*. This insight will awake within him a marvellous wisdom going far beyond all power of description. Such is *pu yen chih chiao* – the teaching without words.

(g) A STORY

About a century ago, a girl called Purple Orchid, being cruelly persecuted by her stepmother, ran off from her home in the city of

Changchou at the age of twelve. After many privations, she was accepted as an inmate of a tumbledown mountain hermitage where five old ladies dwelt far from the world of dust. To her as a youngster fell most of the household chores and she would have felt miserably lonely had not the nature spirits in that vicinity befriended her. She never actually saw them, but the rill where she washed the old ladies' clothes seemed joyously to welcome her presence, as did the stones where she spread the clothes to dry and the trees that sheltered the vegetable garden where she laboured. Her intimacy with these unseen spirits grew so that she shared the happiness of the trees when the sap was rising, of the stream when released from its winter prison of ice, and of the plants when a spell of drought was broken by a shower of rain. Soon she had forgotten the meaning of loneliness.

Though three of the old ladies died off one by one, no one came to replace them, for the times were bad and the mountains had become a haunt of bandits. More than once, wild-looking men descended on the hermitage in search of booty, only to find its scanty stores of rice too full of weevils to be worth carrying away. The only treasure in the place was the person of Purple Orchid, now a winsome girl in her early twenties, but always her invisible friends gave her warning of the danger and provided safe hiding-places unknown to other mortals. Yet there came an evening when three rough fellows forced their way in to demand a night's shelter and discovered Orchid lying in her cell recovering from a brief illness. Shouting to her to get up and cook some supper, they grinned at the thought of further amusement to be had from her later. Seeing her unabashed and ready to return their smiles, they anticipated no resistance when the time came for them to teach her the sport of mandarin ducks.

The two surviving old dames having been ordered to make themselves scarce, the intruders sat down to the meal of coarse vegetables and rice porridge that was all the hermitage had to offer. 'Ah,' cried one of them, 'you are right to smile, Little Sister, for tonight you are going to learn that three lovers have thrice the strength of one.'

While they were busy eating, Purple Orchid tranquilly seated herself cross-legged on a bamboo couch, as though patiently awaiting the pleasures they had promised, but secretly drawing into her body the strength of a great cedar-tree who was her special friend and the present object of her meditation. When the ruffians came for her, it proved no easy matter to lift a girl so seated, her mind out of reach of pain and oblivious to curses, threats and blows; moreover, her slight frame proved to be heavy as a block of cedar wood! At last they managed to stumble with her – legs still crossed in the meditation posture – to her cell, where they dropped her like a wooden statue upon the sleeping-platform and stood back puzzled, sweat dripping from brows already dark with anger. Now one drew a knife and, gesturing with fierce imprecations, ordered the victim to lie down. Receiving no response, he slashed furiously at her leg, but succeeded only in tearing her robe, for the blade slid from her skin as from the bark of a mighty tree. Enraged to the point of madness, he struck and struck again, his companions meanwhile pommelling her with their fists; but they might as well have been dealing with an iron statue of Chung K'uei, Vanquisher of Demons! One by one they grew afraid, awed by the thought that they might be committing sacrilege on the body of a realised immortal. Glancing uneasily at one another, they slunk away.

As for Purple Orchid, she continued to sit rapt, enjoying the sense of power and stillness lent by the cedar tree. Hours passed. When she had returned to an ordinary state of consciousness, a torn and disordered robe was the only evidence that the coming of the ruffians had not been a dream.

Though this story is perhaps fanciful, being founded on a widespread belief in the tutelary spirits said to inhabit rocks, trees, streams and springs, many Taoists assert that the human body can be made invulnerable to weapons by means of practices involving yogic meditation.

4

Cherishing the One (Pao I)

(a) PURPOSE

At the early stages of cultivation, the practice of this yoga leads to stillness, increased vitality and constant awareness of the sublime Tao's interfusion of one's being. At a more advanced stage, it assists in the prolongation of youthful vigour and of one's lifespan. Pursued to the very end, it is a method of attaining the ultimate apotheosis.

(b) INTRODUCTORY

By some masters, Pao I (that is to say 'Cherishing, Guarding or Embracing the One') is believed to be a unique means of achieving the goal without resort to other yogic methods (apart from maintaining a proper diet, breathing and exercising correctly). A traditionally-minded Chinese might be disturbed to find an account of it in a book intended for pupils without access to a teacher who still have much to learn. Yet surely a unique system independent of all others must be suited to people at all stages of development from first to last? Though the instructions given here are not sufficient to guide one through the deeper levels of the yoga, I do believe that great advantage will result from performing it, albeit in a somewhat elementary form.

We have seen that, in an ultimate sense, all things are identical in nature, being manifestations of the same quintessential 'stuff', and that our failure to perceive this is due to our obstinate clinging to a sense of 'I-ness' – a deep-rooted unwillingness to surrender our sense of individuality, even though we may have been assured time and time again that it is illusory. Nevertheless, the fact that we are drawn to the yogic path indicates that something deep within us refuses to be content with the paltry satisfactions offered by the world to those unable to renounce their egocentric viewpoint. It is as though 'a still small voice' were summoning us to higher endeavours. According to Taoist teaching, there exists a drop of unsullied *yang-shên* (*yang*-spirit) within the complicated *yin–yang* structure that one mistakes for 'self'. Indian sages in speaking on an *istadeva* or indwelling deity and Christian mystics in speaking of 'the Christ within' point to the same intuitive recognition that within our being is to be found an unblemished 'drop' of the sublime, undifferentiated Tao.

Cherishing the One means striving to become ever more fully conscious of the presence of this divine link with the ineffable, *and acting accordingly*. The Pao I yoga is intended to promote accomplishment of this aim. Its regular performance will, from the very beginning, help to dispel obstructions to inner stillness and lead towards the dawning of intuitive realisation of our own true nature.

(c) METHOD

Very early in the morning, taking advantage of the powerful currents of *ch'i* circulating at that time, the adept seeks out a quiet place for meditation. It may be the special room or corner he normally uses for that purpose, or else somewhere in the open air where the surroundings are beautiful and, preferably, include a wide vista of hills, plains, sea or sky. A hill-top is ideal, as there should be nothing in the foreground to distract him. Adopting one of the postures and the method of breathing indicated in sections I, B, 2, (b) and (c), he concentrates for a while upon the sensation of breath (and *ch'i*) passing smoothly through the gateway of the nostrils. Next he may embark upon a preliminary meditation which, because its symbolism corresponds to psychic realities known to advanced yogins, forms a good preparation for the main practice.

He visualises his whole body as having been transformed into a beautiful bronze vessel, wide open at the top like a Chinese incense-burner or ritual goblet, standing upon four legs; the open top is bounded by an oblong rectangle of smooth bronze topped at each end by a fixed rectangular handle. Measuring from the tips of the legs to the handles, it is rather taller than it is long. Overhead two long-robed heavenly beings appear, the male bestriding a white tiger (symbol of *yang*, male vitality, the sun, the spiritual realm, etc.), the lady immortal mounted on a green dragon (symbol of *yin*, female vitality, the moon, the terrestrial realm, etc.). From the mouths of their steeds pour fourth streams of dazzling light which mingle in the vessel (i.e.

the adept's body) to form a white elixir. After a while, the white rays are withdrawn and the two immortals fly off to where they vanish in the empyrean. Meanwhile, the elixir rapidly condenses into a small, brightly shining pearl-like object. Thereupon, the bronze vessel regains its human form, but with the dazzling pearl lodged in the psychic centre in the middle of the body parallel to the navel. By concentrating his mind, rolling his eyes several times and breathing deeply, the adept now causes the pearl to rise along the median psychic channel (closely aligned with the spine and reaching the apex of the skull) until it comes to rest in the *ni-huan* cavity which corresponds to the topmost part of the brain. The pearl is in fact the precious drop of spirit that unites the adept to the fount of being.

Now the attention is directed to the main practice, which consists of a meditation on the following lines, though clothed in mental pictures, not in words:

'Here am I, a being at one with my surroundings and yet seemingly bounded by the confines of a body extending only from the top of my skull to the tips of my fingers and toes. Within my head is a sacred cavity containing my most valuable treasure, a shining drop of spirit impervious to contamination, no matter how thickly obscured by dark clouds of delusion. This drop of *yang-shên* is an integral part of me, yet it springs from the very fount of being. Spotless, shining, tiny, it is also infinitely vast, the container of heaven and earth. Herein resides the essence of my selfness, which is not mine at all, but the self of the immeasurable Tao. Herein is the whole meaning of my life, my surest hope of high spiritual attainment. I shall guard full recollection of this treasure by night and day, for it is this which fills me with unlimited vitality and makes me deathless. If I allow it to become so far obscured that it seldom rises to the level of my consciousness, my vital powers will fail with age and, after death, my essence be dissipated and my spirit doomed to gradual dissolution. Such are the dangers of allowing dark obscuring clouds emanating from self-love, inordinate desires, passions and delusion to hide for long the brilliance of this treasure. To the extent that I succeed in piercing their darkness, my *yang-shên* will shine with ever greater brilliance and expand within me until my whole mind and body are filled with its pure substance. Waking or sleeping, I shall cherish recollection of this precious jewel to the utmost of my ability, never allowing it to be far from the surface of my consciousness, never acting in a manner unworthy of it.'

Having thus reflected, the adept should visualise this treasure as a jewel gleaming from within his mind that gradually increases in lustre and expands in size until it fills and shines from every cranny of his body. Expanding still further, it absorbs all his visible surroundings and what lies beyond, reaching to and filling the utmost confines of the universe. At this point, the practised adept will enter into a blissful state (known to Buddhists as *samadhi*) wherein he experiences the perfect identity of beholder, beholding and beheld.

Return to his ordinary state of consciousness should be gradual. In no hurry to move, he should spend a while sitting peacefully as the things about him regain their familiar shapes. Only then should he rise from meditation.

Ideally, he should recollect his 'drop of spirit' at all times, and behave in a manner appropriate to one who is the living repository of so sacred a treasure. This, difficult at first, will become progressively easier until recollection is present in his consciousness even when he is dealing effectively with matters pertaining to the humdrum business of ordinary life. Long before the practice reaches an advanced stage, it will have begun to promote health, vitality, a sense of well-being and stillness of mind, provided that efforts are made to ensure that recollection of the treasure remains close to the threshold of consciousness at all times and that it becomes the main focus of awareness as often as possible.

It has been said by some authorities that frequent practice of the Pao I yoga transforms mind and body so effectively that youthful vigour is prolonged, longevity assured and *physical* deathlessness (meaning life as a Taoist immortal) is achieved. Personally, while not absolutely denying the possibility that such immortals do in some sense exist, I am inclined to think that talk of immortality in this sense results from the inability of the fully realised mystic to convey to others the nature of his intuitive realisation or of the exalted goal to which it leads. One may take the following story in its literal sense if one so chooses, or regard the last paragraph as an allegory hinting at a conclusion more mysterious and subtle than words can tell.

(d) A STORY

A certain scholar called Hsieh in the province of Szech'uan used to spend several hours both morning and evening on contemplating his hidden treasure, besides bringing it to mind whenever he had leisure. When his sons, who privately pooh-poohed this practice as a waste of time, attained to manhood, they were chagrined to observe that more and more strangers took their father for their brother, so little did the passage of time affect his outward appearance. By the time his grandsons were approaching middle age, public astonishment at his still youthful face and figure knew no bounds. The tale was carried to the Emperor who, when Hsieh was already in his early eighties, summoned him to audience. Beholding a vigorous man in the best of health, with black hair, ruddy cheeks and shining eyes, who moved with youthful grace, the Lord of Ten Thousand Years mistook him for an imposter and ordered him to be imprisoned. For a year or two, Hsieh languished forgotten until the Emperor, who had been reading a book on Taoist immortals, summoned him again, thinking: 'After living so long in confinement on poor and scanty food, that impudent fellow is sure to have aged more rapidly than I, whose hair has only recently been touched by autumn frost.' When Hsieh, looking as young as ever, came in and prostrated himself before the Dragon Throne the customary nine times without a hint of effort or fatigue, the Emperor grew thoughtful. Expressing his regret for 'an unfortunate misunderstanding on a previous occasion', he offered the scholar a handsome reward in return for what His Majesty was pleased to term 'the secret of perpetual youth'.

'Sire,' replied Hsieh, 'there is no secret. I have been practising recollection of my *yang-shên* since an early age. That is all there is to it.'

'Will that practice restore lost youth?' inquired the Emperor eagerly.

'Alas, Sire, it can preserve youth but not restore what has already passed away, though it will delay the further onset of old age.' This reply was so displeasing to the August Presence that Hsieh found himself back in prison, where he languished until, following upon the Emperor's death a few months later, he was released by the youngest of the Imperial Princes, brother to the new ruler.

'I am still at the height of my youthful powers,' observed the Prince. 'Kindly impart the means of preserving them.'

'To preserve them', replied the scholar, 'Your Highness must forget about wanting to remain young and just concentrate on Guarding the One, a method I shall be honoured to show you. All else is mere dross.'

Joyfully the young man undertook the practice and it is said that, from about that time until several centuries later, inhabitants of the capital would sometimes come upon two radiant looking persons drinking wine together, one of them apparently a robust fellow in his early fifties, the other a lad in his early twenties. Unfortunately, they would burst out laughing if addressed and promptly vanish.

5

Conservation of the Three Treasures

(a) INTRODUCTORY

The yoga known as the internal alchemy for gathering, nourishing and transmuting the Three Treasures (*ching*, *ch'i*, *shên* and their subtle counterparts) in order to create a spirit body or attain to the grand apotheosis requires a skilful teacher. Thus it is beyond the scope of this book. Nevertheless, all Taoist authorities agree that yogic endeavour at every level requires proper attention to the conservation of those three; never should they be thoughtlessly frittered away.

(b) METHODS OF CONSERVATION

In the male body, seminal fluid is the vehicle of the subtle, invisible energy known as *ching*. This energy, if recklessly expended, is not easily renewable (although, for women, the opposite is true). Being at once a contributing factor to, and an important product of, mental and physical vitality, it must be cherished more lovingly than pearls or jade. Diet, exercise and well regulated sleep all have their part to play, but of even greater consequence is continence. Adepts are not required to abstain from sexual intercourse or to indulge in it only sparingly, but they should carefully regulate seminal emission by stopping short of it on most occasions. Young adepts may perhaps permit release of their semen once a week; as they grow older, the frequence of emission should be gradually reduced; by the age of forty, mind and body should have reached such a stage of serenity that emission is easily avoided altogether. This restriction may seem hard, but it has notable compensations in the form of radiant vitality, both sexual and otherwise.

Ch'i is nourished by yogic breathing (see section I, B, 2, (c)), by exercise and by meditation. Its vehicle in man is breath, its real nature cosmic vitality; it circulates freely throughout sky and earth, but its flow within the body can be obstructed by wrong breathing and/or mental turbulence. From the sky it enters the earth through invisible channels known as 'dragon veins', just as it enters man through the nostrils and pores of the skin, circulating throughout the body along the psychic channels long known to yogins, but invisible to the most powerful microscope, although their existence has now been firmly established even in the West by the science of acupuncture and related practices. Unlike *ching*, it cannot be frittered away because, even in its coarse form, it is not one's own property but a boon freely showered upon all; however, its ingress can be dangerously reduced and its circulation impaired by carelessness. Proper ingress, circulation and purity of *ching* must be maintained by acquiring the habit of correct breathing, rising early in the morning to practise *t'ai chi* or other physical yogic exercises in the open air, abstaining from smoking and avoiding a polluted atmosphere to the extent possible in these days.

Shên is spirit, ordinarily manifested in the form of mental and nervous vitality. It is nourished by meditation, maintaining inner stillness, remaining free from perturbation and, most particularly, avoiding such disruptive passions as anger, envy, jealousy, greed, sadistic joy and lust. (By lust is meant not healthy, creative, inspiring sexual attraction, but turgid passion, obsession, possessive clinging and whatever leads to bitterness rather than joy for either partner or both.) Meditation should be practised frequently, certainly not less than twice a day, and very regularly as regards the times and frequency of sessions. The mind should be guarded day and night from avoidable exposure to the raging winds of passion. This normally requires exercising control over one's choice of companions, reading matter, TV programmes and even thoughts. When thoughts disruptive of serenity arise in the mind, they should not be rigidly suppressed or driven down to remain active below the conscious level; rather they should be watched, examined, recognised for what they are, and quietly but firmly dismissed, as one would dismiss a neighbour's possibly attractive but over-naughty children from one's garden. Conversely, wholesome, creative thoughts should be wooed by every means within one's power (as illustrated by the story that follows). Alcohol, since it quickly loosens control over thoughts and conduct, should be avoided except by those able to enjoy it in strict moderation. The reason why Taoists observe no rigid rules of conduct is that, apart from disliking all forms of rigidity, they do not need them, for their training makes moderation instinctive and joyful.

Shên responds to such forms of nourishment as enjoyment of nature's beauties, contemplation of its processes, fixing the mind upon the sublime Tao and its infinitely varied manifestations, and cultivating deep, dispassionate concentration. Concentration can be stimulated by a wide variety of means; they include poetic composition, calligraphy, painting, music (of an elevating kind), the exercise of any form of skilled craftsmanship, and hobbies such as chess, archery, flower arrangement, gardening, etc. Chess and similar games are good because they require intense concentration, but do not normally arouse a spirit of rivalry. Games of the type that involve gambling, tense excitement, excessive desire for victory, feeling ill will towards one's opponent or partner, etc., should be avoided. Followers of the Way seek for harmony in all things, that their *shên* may remain tranquil, their hearts serene; therefore they keep a watch upon their thoughts and emotions, lest mental and emotional energy be foolishly dissipated.

None of the instructions in this section present great difficulties; many are matters of ordinary common sense; yet they are of great consequence for, unless the Three Treasures are suitably nourished and conserved, all yogic endeavour will be unavailing. Even to acquire spectacular supernormal powers such as levitation, the ability to bend metal objects from a great distance and so on would be yogically useless in the absence of imperturbable serenity.

(c)   A STORY

In the days when the mighty battlemented walls of Peking were still standing and the dwellings surrounded courtyards so full of trees that, viewed from an eminence in summer time, the city looked more like a walled and wooded park than a great metropolis, I came to know a widower who, having sold his modest drugstore business at the age of forty, was fond of describing himself as an idler. Every day, winter and summer, he rose at dawn to perform *t'ai chi* exercises in his courtyard; this done, as he had a daughter and an old woman to look after him, the day stretched unendingly before him, but I never heard him complain that time hung heavily on his hands. Like many Pekingese, he lived closely in accord with the pattern of the seasons and was fond of trees, flowers, birds, singing insects and goldfish.

Around Chinese New Year, which usually falls in February, his little house would be adorned with charming arrangements of narcissus and pebbles in flat earthenware containers, and of sprays of winter-plum blossom standing in antique porcelain vases, but he disdained unseasonable flowers grown in charcoal-heated rooms as being an affront to nature. With the lessening of the cold at the time of the Clear Bright Festival, he would don a well padded robe and go boating on the lakes in the northern part of the city to enjoy, in the company of old friends, the fresh verdure on the willow branches which inspired them to write delicate little poems. These outings would be followed by visits to famous beauty spots in the Western Hills to revel in the burgeoning of spring, from which he would return in a day or two, arms filled with magnolia or branches clothed in fresh spring green with which to make flower arrangements. In May he would spend a lot of time drinking tea with his cronies in one or other of the parks to enjoy the displays of peonies which brought people to the city from a hundred miles around. In June, his courtyard was filled with potted oleanders, pink and white, interspersed with young and slender pomegranate trees; friends would drop in to admire them, or to see the latest additions to the many varieties of goldfish he kept in huge earthenware basins; with the help of a little wine, they would compose poems suggested to them by these things.

During the summer months, the courtyard was roofed in by matting stretched across the tops of poles, and it was too hot to venture out in the middle of the day, but in the late afternoon he loved to stroll on the banks of Peking's many waterways to gaze at the massed lotus rising from a tangle of green leaves that almost hid the water. He liked to fashion fancifully shaped lanterns from these large flat delicately perfumed leaves and, on the Festival of Souls, he was always to be found among the crowds that assembled at night to float frail lotus-leaf craft adorned with lighted candles on the Pei Hai Lake. The onset of autumn was a time for more expeditions to the Western Hills to revel in the scarlet, crimson, yellow, bronze and gold beauty of the maple trees gleaming against the dark foliage of ancient pines and cedars. On the nights of the Mid-Autumn and Double Nine Festivals, he would join a party destined for the top of some small hill to enjoy the brilliant moonlight and the music of flutes or of the silken-stringed *ku ch'in* (a kind of lute) on which they played the plaintive melodies surviving from a far-off age. During the chrysanthemum season, my friend's main living-room was equipped with light wooden stands rising in tiers on which were displayed many dozens of pots of these lovely flowers, which he had personally selected from among a hundred or more varieties to be bought at temple fairs; some were yellow, others bronze, dark red, gold or gleaming white; some had broad petals, others thin and straight or fantastically curling ones; each had its own poetic name, such as dragon beard or golden phoenix. In early winter, he would buy crickets housed in finely made cages of sliced bamboo, whose chirruping enlivened the melancholy evenings. Later, in the season of great cold, he loved to go skating on the Pei Hai Lake, or sit with his friends in a lacquered gallery sipping tea and munching hot dumplings with spiced meat stuffings, meanwhile gazing down at the animated scene on the wide expanse of ice below.

He was often to be found at temple fairs buying flowers or goldfish, which he managed to do at very little cost. Not for him the expensive varieties, for he knew how to choose well among those at which wealthy people would scarcely deign to glance and yet be able to make a fine display for the enjoyment of himself and his friends. A good deal of his time was passed at home reading ancient works, playing melodies on his *ku ch'in*, practising calligraphy, painting delicate likenesses of his favourite trees and flowers, skilfully fashioning all kinds of small objects from wood or bamboo, or playing *wei ch'i* (a kind of chess with 160 pieces on each side) with his daughter, who was an expert player. This sounds an idyllic life, yet he managed to get by on a very modest income. Everything he had was chosen with unerring taste, but very rarely expensive. During the early months of our acquaintance, I thought of him simply as a cheerful, highly gifted dilettante, until one day he spoke by chance of his unremitting cultivation of the Way and his care to nourish and concentrate his *shên*.

'Well,' I said, laughing, 'if your manner of living is what is meant by cultivating the Way, I wonder that a great many more people are not dedicated Taoists. Surely you must be joking?'

'No,' he answered, 'I am as serious about it as a man who smiles at life can be. I perform regular breathing yoga and meditation practice and, apart from those, never cease from nourishing my *shên*. Many people think me frivolous, but my amusements bring me close to nature and make for tranquillity. My life is full and happy, though certainly idle by worldly standards, but I do not dissipate my *shên* by giving way to foolish passions and anxieties. If I live for another hundred years, well and good. If I die tomorrow, well and good, for my mind has been long attuned to the spotless Tao. I call myself an idler because I practise *wu wei* by avoiding activities not consonant with the flow of the Tao. I am in fact quite busy, but nothing I do requires scheming, planning or conflict. You will not see me with clenched teeth or furrowed brow, for I float serenely, borne by nature's current in whatever direction it happens to flow. This is what is known as wandering through life.'

6

Yogic Aspects of I Ching Divination

(a) INTRODUCTORY

The method of using the I Ching (Book of Changes) for divination is set forth in my own and most other translations of that work, so there is no need to repeat the basic instructions here. A good number of people in the West are now familiar with this extraordinary work which, properly used, provides oracles that are most wonderfully fulfilled; but the approach made to it is often too mechanical or too literal, and the point of absurdity has been reached in the United States by the invention of a computer to replace the ancient method of divination with the yarrow stalks or with the (less dependable) coins. The sages who compiled this work some three millennia ago must certainly have relied on intuitive wisdom when writing the texts appended to the hexagrams and moving lines – texts which have won admiration through the ages and more recently impressed the learned C. G. Jung, to say nothing of many other Western intellectuals who regard its oracles as infallible. Therefore, in interpreting the oracles, the promptings of intuitive wisdom should be given precedence over a merely literal or mechanical formulation of the answers. Non-intuitive interpretations may lead to serious errors, for the I Ching is too profound to be properly understood at the ordinary level of consciousness.

(b) METHOD

In casting the yarrow stalks (or, as a poor second best, the coins), the following principles should be meticulously observed:
(i) One must approach the task in a spirit of reverence appropriate to an experience no less awe-inspiring than if one were listening to the

voice of a Supreme Being, for the I Ching's pronouncements, properly interpreted, are just what one would hear if the Tao accorded with the theist conception of God, instead of serenely carrying out its workings heedless of the mortals who pray for guidance. The sages King Wên and Duke Chou attained intuitively to such wisdom that their writings do, in a very real sense, correspond to the transformations of the Tao so accurately as to constitute the nearest possible equivalent to the voice of God.

(ii) In formulating an inquiry, the conscious, logical part of the mind must be used, for the diviner has to consider how best to word it in a manner most appropriate to all the aspects of the situation to be reflected, and to avoid formulations (e.g. either/or questions) unsuited to that method of divination, so he has to be much concerned with verbal precision. Yet, even at this stage, intuition has a part to play. Having reflected at the level of conceptual thought on every facet of the situation prompting the inquiry and arrived at several alternative verbal formulations, he should then strive for mental stillness, banish the content of his thought to the periphery of his mind, and enter into a contemplative state that will allow the best formulation to arise in the stillness as a result of supraconceptual intuition. The inquiry then proceeds with the casting of the yarrow stalks.

(iii) While casting the stalks and dividing them according to the ancient procedure, the diviner should allow his mind to remain in a state of pure receptiveness, so that the fingers and hands may be as free as possible under the circumstances from conscious control and thus able to respond without hindrance to a force that will guide them unerringly. As this may not be easy for beginners, they should practise the manual activity involved in this process again and again until it becomes second nature and can be done correctly with very little in the way of conscious guidance, just as an experienced driver faced by a dire emergency can make the best use of steering-wheel, brake and clutch though there is no time at all to give thought to the matter. The less the conscious mind is involved in manipulation of the stalks, the better. Should fingers and hands begin to jerk like those of a medium in a trance, that is no cause at all for anxiety, but rather an omen of success.

(iv) The I Ching's response to the inquiry is likely to take the form of the texts appended to a hexagram, to one or more moving lines, and to the second hexagram resulting from their movement, all clarified by the nature of the component trigrams, their imagery and so on. Should there be some moving lines and a second hexagram, the appropriate texts should be written down in turn to form a consecutive paragraph. The sentences should then be studied in their relationship to one another and to every aspect of the situation prompting the inquiry. This done, the diviner should cause his mind to become as empty of content as a blank sheet of paper and enter a state of stillness, as in meditation, to await the dawning of intuition. Presently, like a ripple on the still surface of a pond, the correct interpretation of the response will take form within the stillness. If some of the texts are rather long, or if Confucius's commentary is also taken into consideration, it may be best to meditate in this way upon each section of the response in turn, rather than take it as a whole. The method will vary somewhat with circumstances and with individuals; the main thing is to make sure that intuition rather than everyday conceptual thought is made the final vehicle of interpretation.

All the great masters of I Ching divination have used this or a closely analogous method to arrive at their interpretations of its responses, so as to raise their state of consciousness to something like the same level as the state in which King Wên and Duke Chou were inspired to write the texts. The vital importance of resorting to intuitive wisdom holds good, whether one regards the I Ching as the source of divine revelation or prefers what seems to have been C. G. Jung's view, namely that a given response mirrors wisdom present beyond the level of ordinary consciousness in the diviner's own mind.

(c) A STORY

During the Hsien Fêng reign (1851–61) a younger son of Finance Commissioner Pai of Kweichou Province, happening to catch sight of a former schoolmate's sister, felt such an attachment that he was determined to secure her as his wife. As his parents were dead, he was about to send the matchmaker on his own behalf, when it occurred to him to consult the I Ching as a precaution. The response consisted of the hexagram KOU with a moving line in the fifth place and the hexagram TING, which yielded three texts reading: 'Woman wields the power. Do not marry. The medlar leaves wrapping the melon hide its beauty. Something falls from heaven. Sacrifice – supreme success.'

    Being a novice at divination, he looked only for the literal meaning. As a youth long accustomed to sporting in the willow lanes (consorting with courtesans), he was familiar with the term 'melon' as a light-hearted synonym for a certain part of the female anatomy. As the

words 'something falls from heaven' did not seem to fit in with the rest
of the oracle, he ignored them. So his interpretation ran: 'Miss Li is
the sort of woman who would want to rule the roost, so do not marry
her. It is not for you to unveil her melon (perform the nuptial rite with
her). Sacrifice your hope of marrying her and supreme success will
follow' – doubtless in the form of a wife equally beautiful but less
masterful. Yet, so strong was his attachment that he married her in
defiance of the oracle. She turned out to be an admirable wife full of
graceful deference for her husband; so, after a year or two of married
bliss, young Pai decided that the I Ching was a rubbishy sort of book
which had nearly cost him a lifetime of happiness. Once he chanced to
express this opinion vehemently to a group of friends with whom he
was carousing in a wine shop; whereupon an elderly man dressed in
Taoist garb came over to his table and said:

'Forgive me, young sir, for venturing to inquire the reason for your
severe denigration of a book highly revered on every hand.'

Inviting the old man to join his party, Pai laughingly explained the
matter.

'Sir,' replied the Taoist, 'I happen to know the I Ching by heart and
perfectly recall the passages you mentioned. Permit me to ponder
them awhile.' So saying, he became as still as a sage communing with
the Tao, and an atmosphere of austere tranquillity fell upon the
roisterers around them, stilling their idle chatter as effectually as a
peal of thunder. On emerging from this stillness, he continued: 'Truly
you have acted rashly, first by venturing to interpret a book of wisdom
far beyond your understanding; second, by scorning what you
deemed to be its response. Happily the sublime Tao is indifferent to
your impiety. Even so, how can a youth so muddle-headed hope to
escape misfortune? The proper interpretation of the oracle you
received is very different from your own. The injunction not to marry
is entirely negated by the highly auspicious moving line – a case not at
all uncommon, for some moving lines, though by no means all, have
an overriding significance. Note that your spouse's maiden name, Li
(Plum), indicates that the fruit mentioned in the text is to be identified
with her. The correct interpretation of the whole, as applied to your
particular situation at the time, was: "Should you choose to marry at
this time, your wife would be likely to turn out to be a termagant.
Fortunately, your intended bride possesses hidden merits and will
come to you as a rare gift bestowed by heaven. Therefore offer up a
sacrifice in token of gratitude, marry her and you will secure supreme
good fortune." Is not your speaking scornfully of the sacred text a
shameful recompense for heaven's bounty?'

Deeply chastened, Pai offered his apologies, whereat the old man remarked: 'Sir, I perceive you to be a victim of thoughtlessness, rather than a youth of evil disposition. Pray study and take to heart the text appended to the hexagram SHUN and you may yet do well.' To everybody's consternation, the Taoist then vanished – a sure sign of his being an immortal.

Hastening home, Pai looked up the hexagram SHUN and pondered its symbol, 'wood upon wood', which is indicative of unlimited meekness. Thereafter, when things went wrong for him at any time, he accepted these evils tranquilly – a transformation that was one day to save his life. Being appointed at the age of fifty-three as governor of a northern dependency, he once found his way through the mountains barred by a man-eating tiger. He would have drawn his sword and prepared to die in an unequal contest, had not the hexagram SHUN blazed suddenly in his mind. Much affected, he knelt down as though inviting the tiger to have its way with him; but the great beast did no more than caress him with its tongue before shambling off into the twilight. For the rest of his life, Pai lived in accordance with the Way, knowing that nothing in nature will harm one who serenely accepts all things as they come.

7

Healing Yoga

(a) PURPOSES

To heal oneself or others from psychological and physical ills.

(b) INTRODUCTORY

The other practices described throughout this book are given in a largely traditional form, albeit adapted to current conditions in Western countries. With healing, however, adaptation has been taken further. Taoist adepts have always taken keen interest in healing, whether by means of herbal remedies, of which many had a wide knowledge, or of talismans and charms, or by converse with the spirits who can be prevailed upon to enter the bodies of mediums and cause them to write prescriptions while in a state of trance. However one may view this, the remedies were often effective. On the other hand, healing by yogic methods was chiefly employed for dealing with one's own afflictions, rather than those of other people; apart from what can be gleaned from a few stories, I have but little knowledge of the manner in which yogic healing was applied to patients, though there can be no doubt as to its efficacy. In all yogic matters, mind is the king; there are no limits to its powers when properly employed. Here, I have ventured to combine a common Taoist practice (intended for self-healing) with another method derived from Buddhism. The two systems have never been mutually exclusive in China, so borrowings and combinations are entirely in line with tradition.

The Taoist approach to healing is not that of the Christian Scientists, who deplore the supplementary use of medicine. For Taoist yogins, it is not a question of invoking the aid of a divine being who may be supposed to feel displeased by anything less than absolute faith in his intervention, but of drawing upon the infinite power of the Tao, which is present in healer and patient alike, as well as in plants and minerals used for compounding healing drugs. No contradiction is involved in making use simultaneously of spiritual healing and medical treatment. Followers of the Way set no store by praise; if credit for success goes to the medical doctors alone, nobody is the loser.

(c) METHOD OF SELF-HEALING

Preferably in the very early morning the adept, after bodily and ritual cleansing, takes up his meditation posture and performs a simple breathing yoga to quiet his mind and calm any possible disturbances within his body. When free from extraneous thoughts, he concentrates his awareness upon the flow of *ch'i* within himself and throughout earth and sky, reflecting silently:

'My body, though seemingly composed of dense substances, is in reality a transient manifestation of the Tao, not dense but infinitely subtle. It presents no obstacles to the penetration of *ch'i*, which permeates every part of it, entering and leaving by the eight cavities and the pores, and able to pass through sinews, bones and every organ. Obstructions are caused only by mental turmoil or failure to breathe correctly, but now my mind is still, my breathing inaudible, regular and deep yet gentle. I am conscious of *ch'i* flowing through every nook and cranny of my being.' This preliminary meditation should be continued until sensations of lightness, vigour and well-being result.

If the ill to be cured is a psychological flaw, a pressing anxiety or fear, etc., it must now be visualised as a small black cloud hovering at the Dark Gate lying just behind and to either side of the mid-point between the eyes. Should the ill be physical, the cloud is visualised in the affected part of the body and then drawn by the power of mind to settle upon the nearest of five points, namely the Dark Gate behind the eyes, the Ni Huan Cavity just below the apex of the skull, the Heart Centre corresponding to the physical heart but central to the body, the Fire Centre lying at some depth behind the navel, or the Gate of Life and Death at the base of the penis. Ills in the upper limbs should be drawn to the Heart Centre; in the lower limbs, to the Fire Centre.

When the black cloud has reached its appropriate destination, the adept fixes his whole attention upon it, meanwhile allowing nothing to disturb his stillness of mind and body, or the rhythm of his breathing. Then he will become aware of the *ch'i* from within and without playing upon the cloud-like currents of purifying air. Little by little, the cloud will diminish and grow less and less opaque until it vanishes altogether. (Should flashes of white or coloured fire be seen at any time within the Dark Gate, although this is a favourable sign, no particular attention should be paid to it and no feeling of wonder or elation be allowed to mar the stillness.)

The cloud having vanished, the adept remains in a state of absorption for long enough to enjoy the invigorating sensations of lightness and freedom that now occur. Only gradually does he return to his normal state of consciousness and, even then, continues sitting quietly for a minute or two before rising from his seat.

Frequent repetition will make the yoga increasingly effective. Remarkable results are seldom achieved at one sitting, unless by an experienced or naturally gifted healer. Psychological ills can often be put to flight rapidly, sometimes at one sitting – as is the case with anxiety, fear, hysteria, etc. Physical ills are likely to take more time, requiring several sittings; but, should the cause be severe organic damage, then the most that can be hoped for is mitigation of pain and discomfort, as well as of certain symptoms, and a relatively swift recovery to the extent that recovery is possible. Total cure is likely to be beyond the power of an adept of only moderate experience, unless he is endowed with extraordinary gifts. For this reason, one should try to determine at the start of the first session whether the complaint is susceptible to total cure and raise or limit one's aims accordingly. All that is said in this paragraph applies equally, or even more, to the healing of other people.

(d) METHOD OF HEALING OTHERS

Section (c) above should be carefully studied even by those whose purpose is to heal another person, for much that is said there is taken for granted in what follows.

One begins as set forth in the first two paragraphs of (c), except that reflection on the subtle nature of the body and the unobstructed flow of *ch'i* should relate to the patient's body instead of to one's own. The latter, if present, should be sitting or reclining directly in front of the healer; if absent, he should be clearly visualised as being there. The healer next concentrates upon the ill that is to be worked upon, visualising a small black cloud in the patient's head if it is psychological, or in the affected part of his body if physical. By the power of his mind, he causes this cloud to rise in the air and enter the correspond-

ing part of his own body. If, at this stage, the patient's pain or distress communicates itself to him, that is a good sign, but must not be allowed to distract his attention. It will be relatively easy to bear in the full knowledge that it will soon be dissipated by what follows.

The black cloud is now drawn upwards and in through the Dark Gate behind the healer's eyes, not to any other centre, regardless of which part of the patient's body it may have come from. With a powerful wordless aspiration that So-and-so may be quickly cured, the healer contemplates the *ch'i* from within and without his being playing upon the black cloud like currents of healing air until, gradually, the cloud grows less opaque, thins and vanishes. Meanwhile, if the patient is able to do so, he should perform the yoga for self-healing set forth above, to reinforce the healer's powers; in which case both of them may be visited by delicious sensations of lightness and freedom. Returning to an ordinary state of consciousness should be gradual, as in the case of self-healing.

An immediate cure may sometimes be wrought; otherwise, there will surely be some alleviation of pain, distress and other symptoms at each sitting, provided that the yoga is performed conscientiously and the patient co-operates by opening himself up to the healing influence, should he be in a state to do so.

(e) GROUP HEALING

To heal or alleviate one's own psychological ills seldom proves difficult; whereas healing one's physical ills or any ills afflicting another person, apart from temporary hysteria, etc., may prove to be beyond the powers of an adept still new to the practice. On the other hand, group healing – even by novices – is likely to produce striking results from the very beginning; hence this method is to be greatly favoured over the other. The patient is either placed in, or visualised as being in, the centre of a group of from about a dozen to, say, twenty people. These sit cross-legged and facing inwards in a circle. Again, very early in the morning is the best time. Members of the group should have performed the usual cleansing – evacuation of the bowels, bathing, rinsing the mouth and stilling their minds. If there has been a gap between their doing these things and the beginning of the healing session, their minds should have been kept tranquil, free from turbulence or anxiety, and occupied with pleasant, dispassionate, uplifting thoughts. When they have taken up position in the circle, each stage of the yoga should be very carefully explained to them in advance. This done, the group performs the healing yoga set forth above in section (d), commencing of course with controlled breathing and stilling of the mind. The patient's co-operation should, if possible, be sought; either he should remain tranquil and open himself up to the healing influences or, better still, perform self-healing yoga while the others strive to heal him.

Besides the group leader – preferably an experienced adept or healer, whose task it is to make sure that everybody knows exactly what to do – it may be useful to have a time-keeper, as different members of the group will be apt to devote varying lengths of time to each stage of the yoga. His function would be to indicate when a new stage should be jointly embarked upon, by softly striking two resonant blocks of wood together at the junctures marked by an asterisk in the following summary; but the sound should not be loud enough to startle or distract; and, if he is taking part himself in the yogic practice, he should wait a little after concluding each stage in his own mind, to allow reasonable time for others to catch up. The rest of the group should each continue with the appropriate stage until the wood-blocks sound, even after they feel ready to embark upon the next stage. Except during group healing, however, no time limits are to be observed, for an adept working alone must decide for himself when a stage has been successfully completed.

(f)   SUMMARY OF THE PRACTICES

Cleansing
Breath control and stilling of the mind (5–10 minutes)
* Reflection on the subtle nature of the body and flow of *ch'i* (5–10 minutes)
* Visualisation of the black cloud and drawing it into oneself (2 minutes)
* Dissipation of the cloud and enjoyment of the sensations of lightness and freedom (10–20 minutes)
* Gradual return to a normal state of consciousness (3 minutes)
* Quietly sitting before rising (2 minutes)

(g)   A STORY

Prefect Chin came from a distinguished line of scholars who had held important posts throughout the Empire for four generations. His wife having failed to bear the son needed to continue this line, he took three concubines in turn, but they too bore him only daughters until the youngest at last conceived a son whose birth cost her her life. This boy, Chin Hung, though inclined to be weakly, was handsome and very good at his studies. He received an excellent education and showed satisfactory academic promise, but he was a frequent prey to fits of melancholy, had an unreasoning fear of the demon-haunted night, and sometimes trembled and gibbered like an idiot boy, so obsessed was he by the thought of having brought about his mother's death. Many a doctor and tutor was brought to the house with instructions to cure him, for his mental state seemed likely to impair his performance in the state examinations on which hung all hope of advancement leading to a distinguished career. Finding their efforts vain, some attributed his condition to the malevolence of demons, while others declared that the servants must have filled his head with their ignorant chatter about demons, ghosts, sprites and suchlike, until his *shên* was disturbed by morbid fancies.

At the age of sixteen, while studying at the nearby Academy of Austere Virtue, he conceived an attachment for Hsiao Mao (Kitten), the fifteen-year-old daughter of the overseer of the family mansion, who had just entered upon her duties as maid to one of his sisters. The affair flourished in secret for a few months, the lovers holding nightly tryst in a garden pavilion rarely frequented after dark, for the boy's fear of demons proved no match for his youthful passion. But, as the proverb says, 'Heaven sees all', and in course of time their liaison came to light. The overseer, son and grandson of family retainers, could not be banished from the mansion, but he was prevailed upon to agree to his daughter's being sent away to serve a cousin of the Chin family in distant Yangchow. First, he gave her a good beating for leading the poor young master astray. On the night before she was due to leave, the lovers snatched a final meeting in a bamboo grove bordering the handsomely landscaped garden, there being some rocks on which to sit among the graceful fronds. Weeping copiously, Kitten declared:

'Three times the goddess Niang Niang came to me in a dream. Smiling, she told me all will be well. How can that be, unless we run off together?'

'Impossible!' cried Chin Hung, mingling his tears with hers. 'Could I survive the awful knowledge of having murdered *both* my parents? My honoured father's rage and sorrow at having his hopes dashed by my deliberate act would surely kill him. Who knows how fearfully we should be punished by fate?'

'Then we must part, Young Master', murmured Kitten dolefully. 'Still, before I go there's something I can do for you. The goddess showed me how. Ask no questions. Just sit down on that flat rock. Empty your mind. Stay still. Do nothing.'

To please her, Chin Hung complied. Seating herself cross-legged on another rock, she seemed to go off into a trance. So still were they that the wheeling moths settled on their garments and once a bat came to rest on Chin Hung's shoulder. Presently a beam of light seemed to issue from between Hsiao Mao's eyes and enter him, growing brighter and brighter as it streamed through the Dark Gate behind his forehead. At any other time, this would have made him shiver with fear, but now he was determined to please her and soon found himself strangely at peace. The light seemed to coagulate in the Dark Gate, then to melt again and send a shining white stream down the centre of his body to throat, heart, navel and the Gate of Life and Death. Smaller streams, fanning out to either side, spread to every part of his being. Glancing down, he perceived that he now resembled a crystal statue filled with white fire that illumined the bamboos and rocks around him and made Hsiao Mao look radiant as the goddess Niang Niang! When the beam from her forehead was withdrawn, the light within him slowly dimmed until the two of them returned to being dark shapes barely visible to each other. The lovers were smiling as they stood cheek to cheek in farewell, but they shed more tears when the crowing of a cock warned them to slip back to their separate quarters in the house before sleepy maids emerged to tend the stoves. Later that morning, a cart driven by Kitten's brother took her and her modest luggage to the river bank where a vessel was just about to cast off for the voyage to Yangchow.

The old prefect's fears that his son would be dazed out of his wits by the parting were not fulfilled. Certainly the boy was cast down for a few days, but he soon recovered and, thereafter, never once exhibited the symptoms of an unbalanced mind that had troubled him for years. On the contrary, he became quietly self-possessed and even more studious than before, went confidently to each round of examinations during the following years and, in his mid-twenties, received the supreme scholastic honour of a Han Lin degree. Returning home from the capital in triumph, he hurried in to prostrate himself before his august parent and, after a suitable interval, acquainted the old man with all that had passed during his final tryst with Hsiao Mao.

Not altogether pleased, the former prefect murmured thoughtfully: 'The decrees of High Heaven are so often inscrutable that one does not commit the folly of turning the head to left and right when one of them happens to be clear. Yet we cannot with impunity break off the engagement I made for you with the second daughter of Magistrate Tu. It will be best to take that little minx, Kitten, as a minor wife. To forestall objections, I will acquaint the Tu family with the circumstances. They will not expect you to reject a mandate from Heaven.'

Hsiao Mao served the senior wife respectfully until the latter's untimely death during a smallpox epidemic some six years later. Thereafter, the old prefect having gone to rejoin his ancestors meanwhile, the surviving wife led Chin Hung into the mountains to cultivate the Way.

8

Supportive Practices

(a) PURPOSE

To achieve through beauty in all its forms a heightened insight into reality as a preparation for, and stimulus to, intuitive experience of man's intimate relationship with the sublime Tao.

(b) INTRODUCTORY

The Tao is often conceived of as a shining, intangible non-substance of infinite extent creating from its own being the innumerable wavelike forms that Lao-tzû calls the myriad objects. All are transitory and forever in a state of growth or decline; all have the capability of becoming one another since, ultimately, they are never apart from or different in nature from the whole. Thus man and his environment are indivisible. Taoist painters hint at this mystery in skilful ways, often by delineating mountains, clouds and watery expanses as shadowy masses suggestive of endless interchange and transformation; or by painting in tiny human figures as integral but very far from dominating parts of a landscape; or, conversely, by giving immense significance to things ordinarily deemed unworthy of notice, such as a patch of coarse scrub-grass in the foreground of an otherwise undifferentiated and limitless expanse of snow. Or they may depict lifelike forms issuing from what we call inanimate matter, perhaps rocks seemingly caught in the very act of giving birth to craggy birds, animals or monsters. Always the implication is that every entity, organic or otherwise, is imbued with life-force and an embodiment of the Tao,

---

[1]For the full texts of the poems from which these extracts are taken, see my earlier work, *Taoism: the Search for Immortality*.

from which none has ever been truly apart or lastingly differentiated. In the words of Lü Yen, 'Green mountains are white clouds in a passing transformation.'[1] Pai Yü Ch'an's lines 'Swiftly runs the stream, tinged by fragrant grasses; the ancient pines are dyed with the bluish tint of distant mountains'[1] hint at the same mysterious interpenetration of apparently diverse objects.

(c) CREATIVE POETRY

Taoists regard poetry as an admirable medium for expressing man's innate kinship with nature. Their verses are rich in references to sights and sounds which reinforce this feeling. Floating clouds signify the freedom of a sage who has shed the gross delusion of solidity and apartness, thus liberating himself from compulsion to go anywhere in particular or do anything but steer his barque as it is borne joyously along on the tide of circumstance. Phrases like 'the music of falling rain' suggest that joy and beauty are to be found even in those natural phenomena which an unperceptive person may regard as inimical to the plans of mice and men – how much more so, that exquisite phrase 'the *companionable* roar of a cliff-dwelling tiger'![1] The elemental sounds produced by the percussion instruments employed by recluses to punctuate their chanting, such as a stone bell or a hollowed block of resonant wood, are esteemed because, apart from their association with ancient rituals, they resemble sounds produced by nature without the instrumentality of man. As with romantic poetry in all languages, Taoist poems are replete with phrases now considered trite, such as 'radiant moonlight', 'coral clouds', 'spring blossom', 'autumnal splendour', 'snowy boughs', 'the creak of feathery bamboos', 'the soughing of the wind among the pines' and so forth. I never tire of them, because they are marvellously evocative of things I love and very often used to bring to mind the hidden mystery with which the whole of nature is interfused.

I know from experience that there are sights and sounds which, upon occasion, act on a mind attuned to nature like a powerful incantation: a sudden glimpse of dripping mossy stones lit by dappled sunshine, or the sigh of wind amidst the reeds lining the margin of a pool may, as it were, twitch aside a veil, affording a breath-catching intimation of the unearthly loveliness underlying the sometimes humdrum world apparent to our sadly inadequate senses. In a brief flash of ecstasy, the holiness and stupendous significance of what we often take for trivial phenomena stands revealed. Ah, the joy of such moments! This *satori*-like experience is all the more intense for being unlooked-for. Meditation, contemplation of nature and immersing ourselves in Taoist art and poetry are all ways of heightening perception of the hidden glory, of meaning beyond meaning beyond meaning. The mind needs to be prepared by attaining insights into the truth that the Tao, formless and without dimensions, is *fully* present in the tip of a blade of grass or any other microscopic object no less than in the great firmament above and below the world. Without such insights, the twitching aside of the veil might be too fleeting to impinge upon our consciousness at all, and great would be our loss.

To penetrate to the inner meaning of Taoist art and poetry, or to be able to create paintings and poems even lightly imbued with that meaning, is a valuable part of yogic training. Being no painter, I shall confine myself to describing how the writing of simple nature poems can be used as a form of yoga.

First it is necessary to become steeped in Taoist poetry, whether in the original or in translation, so as to attain a proper perspective in which to view nature through Taoist eyes. It is good to allow full rein to fancy, paying homage to rocks and streams and trees and pools by accepting that they are peopled by nature spirits, those shy beings whom one may learn to see simply by believing in them. Who would not be glad to encounter, as our ancestors often did, a forest nymph peeping at him from behind the trees or a smiling old man, beard down to his knees, emerging from a rainbow-sprayed waterfall? Myth opens more doors than science to perception of the nature of being, for the latter deals only with the material world and has nothing to say of those levels of truth that are perceived only when the illusion of gross materiality has been *seen through*. To insist that nature spirits do not exist may be absolutely right in one sense, and yet perhaps quite wrong in another. Such fanciful concepts acquire new dimensions once it is realised that 'the stuff of the universe is mindstuff', that is to say more closely analogous to pure consciousness than to any other definable 'substance'; for then thoughts, dreams, reveries take on a reality not essentially different from that of rocks and trees. Indeed, dream forms are *more* real to the dreamer than flesh-and-blood forms to a waking man when not actually in his presence; for the former give rise to sensations of seeing, hearing and, sometimes, of touch, which an absent person or object obviously cannot do. The worth of poetic fancy to those who seek to penetrate beyond gross materiality would be hard to exaggerate.

Besides reading poems that have come down through the ages, preparation for writing Taoistic poems of one's own, as a means of deepening perception of the nature of reality, includes wandering often amidst the solitude of woods and hills. By all means let the fancy people the solitude with invisible nature spirits – some benevolent, others mischievous or hostile to intruders – for these beings may occasionally manifest themselves to those with eyes to see. Besides, it is a means of cultivating that attitude of reverential awe for the holiness of the natural environment which modern man has lost. Who would wantonly cut down a tree believed to be the habitation of a spirit? That a wanderer in a reverent state of mind may occasionally encounter nature spirits, and be touched by the awesomeness of being on the fringes of a mystery, does not imply that they are real in a narrowly scientific sense – but then, indeed, there is nothing in the universe than can properly be described as real in itself, all thoughts and objects being manifestations of the formless Tao. Conversely, should he fail to encounter any, that would not mean that none are peering at him from their lichened grottoes and leafy boles!

One should be alert, too, to nuances of atmosphere, to the interplay of movement and stillness all around. Even the most insignificant sights and sounds are worthy of attention; for, unless alertness is keen, the veil I have spoken of may be twitched aside in vain and one of life's most blissful experiences forgone. Sounds, no less than sights, should be savoured to the full – the tinkle or roar of running water, the scurrying of small creatures, the songs of birds and insects, the soughing of the breeze, the rhythmic blows of a woodman's axe or the tapping of a woodpecker, the lowing of distant cattle, the wind-borne cries of children at play in a valley far below. In China, one used to hear at times the solemn reverberations of a temple gong, or the bok-bok-bok of a hermit's wooden 'fish-drum'. All alike are nature's voice – the voice of the Tao!

Alertness is vital, but the mind should not become involved in making needless distinctions. Primroses shining in the sunlight are primroses shining in the sunlight. What can their genus, species, anatomic detail and method of procreation matter in comparison to the joy they bring? Their comeliness, their lovely hues varying with the play of light on leaves and petals, their essential 'rightness' in that setting make them unique – a sight never to be repeated in exactly the same form. The nature poet esteems immediacy of experience, not second-hand knowledge derived from books. Furthermore, no matter how enticing the beauty of the flowers, he will not be tempted to pluck them; unless driven by hunger to eat them, why should he requite nature's bounty by destroying its precious gift?

The sight of sailing clouds leads to musing upon the transience and mutability of forms, so swiftly do castles, cliffs and islands in the sky dissolve, merge and form new shapes, thus mirroring the changes that occur on different time-scales throughout the whole of nature's realm. Even mountains are ephemeral by the standards of eternity. A vista of hills and clouds, or clouds and sea, is a reminder that phenomena, being wholly composed of the pure non-substance of the Tao, melt freely into one another. The sequence cloud–rain–lake–river–sea– rising moisture–cloud is but a rather easily observable instance of the principle that causes mountains to sink into the sea, or a sea-shell-strewn ocean bed to be lifted and become a majestic mountain chain.

Such musings and reflections, stored in the mind for later use, are the very stuff of Taoist painting and poetry. Creating either of these is a kind of yoga in itself. By no means everyone is a gifted artist or poet; our attempts to capure beauty in brush strokes or poems may excite the laughter of the world, but this matters very little, for it is the action of creating that has a yogic value. Moreover, creative works, born of intuition, of communion with nature and meditation on the sublime Tao, no matter how trifling their workmanship and technical accomplishment, will enshrine the quintessence of the doctrine of Not Two. During the act of creation, the mind will soar above the dualism of mind and matter, this and that, self and other, without danger of alighting in the mire of a vague and misleading 'all is one, nothing matters' philosophy. All is not one; all is not many; one is one; many are many; one and many are Not Two; all is Not Two.

This teaching, so hard to encompass in words or thoughts, is the fruit of mystical intuition which makes it laughably easy to comprehend; and mystical intuition is most often arrived at during meditation or when the mind is concentrated upon Tao-inspired creativity. An adept does not seek to impress the world by his poems, painting or calligraphy, but to penetrate more deeply into his own mind while creating them, and thus come closer to intuiting the nature of the Tao. Technical ineptitude simply does not matter. After all, there are always waste-paper baskets for use when the joyous moments of creativity are passed.

Here is a poem somewhat in the Chinese manner as regards content, though naturally different in metrical form as Chinese forms are hardly possible to reproduce in English. I wrote it in the garden of a villa on Mount Tamalpias, overlooking San Francisco Bay. The scene poignantly reminded me of China's Chiang Nan region, where so many Taoist hermitages are situated; even the great bridge leading across to Berkeley helped the illusion as, from that distance, it resembled a modest structure of bamboo.

The pines are singing of Chiang Nan,
So distant, yet before my eyes.
A bamboo bridge hangs motionless
As though to flout the breeze's whims.

At dusk, a myriad fallen stars
Bestrew the further shore with gems
And homing pleasure craft, like moths,
Flit stealthily across the bay.

A strange bird gigglingly inquires
With avian impertinence:
'Why did you fly across the world
To see what lay so near at hand?'

This is decidedly not great poetry, but it has caught some gleams of Taoist wisdom. Chiang Nan with its pine-trees, waterways and green rolling hills, so far away and yet right there before my eyes, recalls the Tao stretching out a billion trillion miles beyond me and yet nearer than my nose is to my lips. A tremendous steel and concrete causeway is transmuted by distance into a rustic bamboo bridge, just as great cities and parklands are transformed into wildernesses, or wildernesses into lush forests by the action of the Tao. Electric lights *are* stars to eyes that see them so. Wherever man may travel, he never leaves home, for his true home is the measureless ocean of the Tao in which he is born, lives and dies.

(d) THE RHYMING GAME

A pleasant recreation which also serves as an adjunct to cultivation of the Way is a rhyming game, which is especially appropriate to such occasions as when friends assemble on a moon terrace to enjoy a vista of moonlit mountains and plains and to eat, drink, laugh and play as they bathe in a soft, mind-intoxicating radiance. However, a garden or any lovely place will do. It starts with somebody improvising a line of poetry, usually suggested by his surroundings, and inviting his companions to compose, each within an agreed length of time, lines matching it in content, metre and rhyme. Failure to respond in time is penalised by the culprit's having to drain a small cupful of wine and lose his turn, it being assumed that no one is so thirsty or dead to poetic feeling that he would fail voluntarily. The game is more difficult to play in English than in Chinese, because there are fewer rhymes and too many tiresome 'a's, 'the's, '—ing's and '—ed's which take up room that could otherwise be used for more significant syllables, thereby reducing the volume of meaning that can be contained in each line; so it is best to allow a rather loose rhythm and not be too finicky about rhyme. It is thought, not form, that matters. That is how I play the game on the rare occasions when I can inveigle some friends into trying their hand at it. The opening line should be one that is easy to match; otherwise the game becomes impossible. There are no winners or losers, so one hopes others will be successful and feels no sense of triumph in their failure. Verses improvised in this way – at least in a European language with its complicated grammar – are very rarely of high quality, but they often reflect sudden flashes of insight into the nature of the Tao. If not inspiring, they may at least be inspired.

Once I was picnicking with some friends in the garden of a Burmese-style temple, with perhaps a hundred wind bells depending from its eaves, built on the apex of a small hill overlooking the mountain-girt city of Maesarieng in northern Thailand. The sun had set in a blaze of colour behind the western mountains and a gibbous moon shone down on the stark white, gracefully tapering pagodas. While I was filling the wine cups, someone forestalled me by declaiming *'White moonlight gleaming on these towers'*, which I followed up with *'Demands a toast to radiant beauty'*. The third player was so slow in continuing the poem that the fourth called *'Unless you quickly improvise'*, whereat the third responded wryly *'To drink it will become my duty'*.

Considering that the other three had played this game only once before, I thought this merry opening very good. Laughing heartily, everyone lost the feeling of being tongue-tied. Presently I intoned *'Find words now to describe the Tao'*. Just in time, the person on my left retorted *'Too subtle! It eludes our grasp'*. There followed such a long pause that someone, remembering the previous poem, cried *'Raise your cup. Prepare to drink'*, bringing the triumphant response *'What else then will my fingers clasp?'* The lady in our group had hit the nail on the head, recognising that the Tao is what is, whether sun and moon or wine cup. She told us that her sudden recollection of an analogous Zen *koan* had inspired that brilliant line.

When the game is played by people familiar with Zen and Taoist ways of thinking, such flashes of insight are not infrequent, which is why whole verses are occasionally produced with scarcely any hesitation at all. Once some friends were dining in my garden, where there is a six-foot white pagoda flanked by porcelain lions. After one or two

stillborn attempts, the following verse flashed out with hardly a pause
between the lines:

> *White tower, blue lions, grass encircled,*
> *A green bronze censor, incense lit;*
> *The Tao pays heed to none of these –*
> *Yet they are naught apart from it!*

Admirable! Though technically no masterpiece, the verse exactly
expresses what Lao-tzû meant by saying that the Tao 'requires no
recompense' for its benificence, being unconcerned with man;
whereas man, his possessions and whole environment have no existence outside the being of the Tao.

Should verses thus composed prove very faulty as to composition,
rhythm or rhyme, they can of course be polished later, though not
without risk of losing spontaneity. Here is an example of overpolish-
ing; seeking to improve the quality of the verse, I strayed too far from
the sense of the original:

> *White moonlight gleaming on these towers*
> *Demands a toast to radiant beauty.*
> *Unless you quickly improvise,*
> *To drink it will become your* duty.*

(*Necessarily changed from 'my')

> *Bathed in a sea of pearly radiance,*
> *These gleaming pinnacles*
> *Recall the icy bastions that guard*
> *The palace of the Goddess of the Moon.*
> *Inspired, we woo this chaste and lovely being*
> *With offerings of poesy and wine.*

On the other hand, there is something to be said for the amendment
of the second poem, though personally I prefer the original.

> *Find words now to describe the Tao.*
> *Too subtle! It eludes our grasp.*
> *But when I raise my cup to drink**
> *What else then will my fingers clasp?*

(*Necessary change)

> *Mere words cannot define the Tao;*
> *Its subtlety eludes our grasp.*
> *And yet it's what I'm holding now,*
> *Being everything our fingers clasp.*

(e) MOONLIGHT AND FLUTES

I well recall the enchantment of moonlight picnics held on certain
feast days, such as the Clear Bright Festival in early spring, the
Birthday of the Moon Goddess in mid-autumn and the Hill Climb-
ing Festival that falls about a month later. I do not see why Westerners with no moon calendar to guide them should not enjoy
themselves Taoistically on any moonlit night, if the weather is
propitious and a good place (even a rooftop) can be found for
viewing sky and earth. On the birthday of Chang Ô, the Moon
Goddess, it was usual to make offerings of large flat moon-shaped
cakes, glistening white in colour, being confections of white flour
or ground rice and sugar. These would be placed on a suitably
decorated table facing the moon, perhaps with representations of
the Goddess and of the jade rabbit and jade toad which, sharing her
glittering ice palace, are forever engaged in the task of compounding a store of the elixir of immortality. If all this is thought too
fanciful, people can omit the ceremony and honour her simply by
enjoying themselves. After a picnic dinner accompanied by wine,
there can be demonstrations of skill in the defensive arts, *t'ai chi,
judo, kung fu, taekwando* all being appropriate because embodying
Taoist principles; or one can play the rhyming game, or just
declaim a few old poems, but at all costs someone should be found
to play beautifully on a flute, preferably the long lacquered bamboo
kind that is carried in a silken sheath strapped to one's back, but
any kind of flute will do very well. The sound of this instrument
combines so deliciously with moonlight that even a flautist of moderate talent can arouse his friends to ecstasy. The high sweet notes
and soft white radiance affect one so poignantly that the mind is
carried away into a faery realm peopled by sages and immortals.
One almost expects to see the Longevity Fairy bestriding a giant
crane, his snowy beard, long silken sleeves and robe streaming
behind him as he soars above the earth. Who knows that the lovely
notes will not summon Han Hsiang-tzû, the exquisite, forever
youthful flautist whose music can charm even dragons from the
clouds and rivers, or unicorns from the forest, to come and add
their many-coloured splendour to the scene? Even if nothing out of
the ordinary should happen, moonlight and the music of flutes
have a strange affinity that leads those present to heightened states
of consciousness like those experienced by sages skilled in meditation. As a background to contemplation of the mystery of being,
the sublimity of the Tao, they are unrivalled.

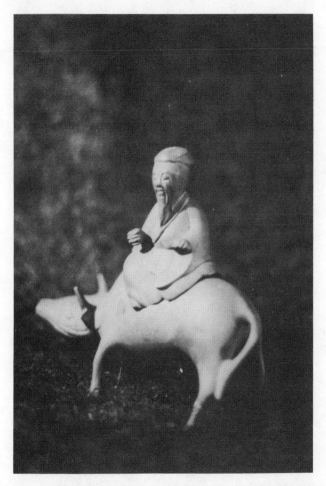

Lao-tzû riding on an ox (*author's collection*)

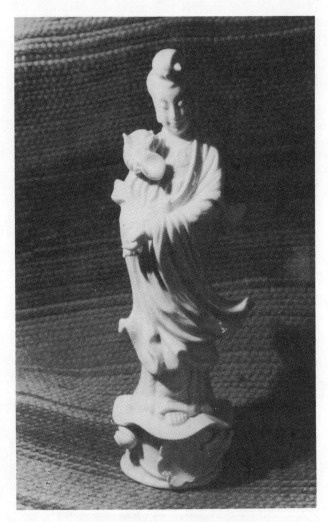

Kuan Yin (*author's collection*)

(f) EXPLORING HIDDEN BEAUTY

Taoists never tire of gazing at rocks and mountain crests with shapes suggestive of living beings emerging from an amorphous mass, as though titans, dragons, humans, animals and birds were taking form before their eyes, being born from the undifferentiated non-substance of the Tao. All over China, names such as Lion Peak, Nine Dragon Mountain, Phoenix Rock, Tiger Stalking Deer Ridge bear witness to the special kind of perception that acquaintance with Taoist mysteries evokes. To wander through or gaze at mountains while allowing the imagination full play is an absorbing pastime and very valuable as a reinforcement to yogic understanding of the nature of being, for it soon appears that the division of natural objects into animate and inanimate has only relative validity; certain rocks emanate such a haunting atmosphere that one cannot doubt their awareness of the presence of an intruder, whether it is an atmosphere that draws one to linger in the vicinity or so awe-inspiring as to cause an urge to hurry on. At the deeper levels of understanding, it is apparent that every atom of the universe is imbued with life, being inseparable from the living Tao.

A no less fruitful practice is to gaze at vistas of cloud, at patterns formed by the grain of certain woods or – as every small child used to know before coal and wood fires were banished – at the glowing embers of a fire. Beauty can be found even at the heart of ugliness. The grain of a cheap wooden door, peeling whitewash on a bathroom window, a patch of damp on the concrete wall of a prison, drops of oil spreading out in a filthy puddle, discoloration on a plaster ceiling – in these one can often discern all kinds of lovely beings, beguiling gnomes and fairies, knights in armour, seductive maidens, smiling goddesses, amusingly baleful demons, Taoist immortals, Arabian Nights viziers, Christian monks and nuns, Byzantine dignitaries. Indeed there is no end to their variety. Besides beings, the grain of wood or patches of discoloured concrete also yield chains of mountains, dense forests, lonely cedars – again there is no end. One may live in a hovel and yet be surrounded by beauty, if only one has eyes to see.

(g) TAILPIECE: PROPHETIC DREAMS

Here I am treading on only slightly familiar ground and am not sure of my bearings. In certain Taoist hermitages can be found a building set apart for dreaming auspicious dreams, but this is a practice pertaining rather to the ancient Chinese folk religion, with whose hundreds and thousands of deities I have only a nodding acquaintance. There is also such a thing as yogic dreaming, but I have received no instruction in that art. I have added this tailpiece for two reasons. The first is that, as Taoism at its popular level came to be closely entwined with the folk religion, it seems fitting to include one of the resulting practices in this book. Second, I myself once had what was believed to be an encounter with an immortal in a specially induced dream. As related fully in my book, *The Secret and Sublime*, a certain Taoist recluse arranged for me (by what means I do not know) to encounter in a dream a being called Lü Tung-pin, who is pre-eminent among a group known as the Eight Immortals. That very night, I dreamed of this handsome, bearded swordsman, master of *kung fu* and magic arts, who favoured me with what must surely have been a fateful message touching my own future as a cultivator of the Way. Though he appeared easygoing and laughed a lot, being doubtless amused that a foreign devil should have sought him out, he seemed serious about what he had to say. On waking foolishly elated, I dwelt upon the visual aspects of the dream so dotingly that, by breakfast time, I had actually forgotten the greater part of what the immortal had been graciously pleased to tell me! My hosts, though too courteous to chide me severely, must have been aghast at my casual treatment of sacred matters!

Having found the Taoist recluses I met to be, by and large, highly intelligent people, I have never scoffed at those of their beliefs that strike me as far-fetched or otherwise hard to accept. In seeking to penetrate to the roots of another culture, it is best to be open-minded and more inclined to accept than reject what one is told. There is always much that a newcomer is not qualified to understand, much less judge; moreover, such an attitude wins the trust of people who would certainly keep many wonderful things secret if they feared their sacred mysteries would be scorned. That is why it is often difficult for scholars doing research into such matters to penetrate much below the surface. Besides, people educated in the modern West (most certainly including me) are often hindered by the nature of our education from accepting what may indeed be true, if its truth lies outside the scope of scientific investigation.

One method of inducing auspicious or prophetic dreams is thus. One procures a likeness of one of the Eight Immortals, or of some similar being such as the bald, snowy-bearded Longevity Fairy, whose symbols are a deer, peach or peachwood staff and a crane. A picture or statue of Lao-tzû might be even more appropriate. All these beings figure so prominently in Chinese art that it is no longer difficult to acquire something suitable in the West. The Chinatowns of San Francisco, New York, Boston, Chicago, Vancouver, Toronto, etc., all have them. Whether or not one quite believes in them as objectively existing supernatural beings, there is something mysterious about the responses received by those who ceremoniously invoke their aid. The picture or image should be placed close to the head of the bed where one proposes to dream, never near the foot and never at a lower level than one's breast when standing erect. At bedtime, light a stick of incense, bow reverently, and politely request the favour of a prophetic dream. Then lie down on the right side with the right hand placed palm upward between one's face and the pillow beneath it. Go to sleep as quickly as possible without allowing too many extraneous thoughts and reveries to intervene. If they do, when at last sleep does seem near, repeat the request while lying down. To get up and light more incense might drive sleep away. If a light-switch, paper and pencil are placed within easy reach, the dream can be recorded at the moment of waking, while the details are still vivid and any words spoken can be clearly remembered.

To behold in a dream the being to whom one's petition has been addressed is believed by my Chinese friends to be a mark of signal favour; to hear that being speak is even more auspicious, though perhaps hard to accomplish without the aid of a Taoist skilled in such matters. Supposing that neither of these things happens, one should carefully transcribe the first coherent and clearly defined dream to come that night. It is said that this dream, rightly interpreted, is sure to yield a message of great consequence to the dreamer. Should several sleepers obtain striking responses in one particular house or room, rather than another, that would be an indication that the place is particularly propitious for this practice.

As I have said, I am skating on thin ice here. I do not know the territory and have merely retailed what Chinese friends have told me. I can neither guarantee success nor offer advice as to how such dreams should be interpreted; but an experiment might prove worthwhile. One or two failures need not be taken to mean that success is impossible.

Soon after writing this paragraph, I tried the experiment myself, with a result that was certainly not negligible, but rather too embarrassing to recount.

Part II *Mahayana Buddhist Theory and Practice*

A THEORY

1

The
Philosophic Base

(a) NOT TWO

Mahayana Buddhism is a system offering many different means of cultivating the Way, some suited to people with simple goals, others requiring immense and unflagging dedication.

By no means all Buddhists are mentally and spiritually equipped to grasp the more profound ideas developed in the Mahayana sutras; and, even among those able to grasp them, the sense of urgency and divine discontent that drives some wise people to attempt speedy attainment of the ultimate goal – Enlightenment – are confined to a small proportion of the whole. The majority of Buddhists are content to learn how to live wisely, happily and compassionately in the present life, in the belief that such conduct will ensure an auspicious rebirth in circumstances better suited to entering upon the higher levels of the Way. Well, even that relatively limited aim is well worth pursuing, besides involving practices that will constitute a sound preparation for going much further, whether in this life or another. Some of these practices are described in the following pages; they will be found speedily effective in improving the quality of life in the Here and Now, the emphasis being on things *to be* and *to do*; but, as most of them can also be used for the achievement of more exalted aims, I have thought it best to begin by touching upon the subtle and not very easily understandable philosophic base.

Comprehension of this philosophic base is of course essential for yogic giants who (like those Taoists dedicated to achieving the supreme apotheosis, Return to the Source) seek attainment of Enlightenment in this very life. That is a truly stupendous task requiring unremitting zeal night and day for many years on end. Enlightenment entails passing beyond the confines of relative truth as reported by our senses, taking a great leap into the realm of the void which can be apprehended only through mystical intuition of a very high order, returning thence to the realm of form (now seen in a new perspective), and penetrating the mystery of the Not Two. This is the only road to the state of Nirvana in which all dualistic categories – existence and non-existence, eternal life and extinction, self and other – are transcended.

The Enlightened One (the Buddha) made no assertions concerning Nirvana. To questions such as whether it implies eternal life or extinction, he would reply 'Not that, not that', his purpose being neither to mystify nor hold something back, but simply to signify that no meaningful assertions *can* be made, even by one who has experienced it, about a state of being so exalted as to be void of attributes, qualities or distinguishing characteristics of any kind whatsoever. Even to say that beings continue to exist or cease to exist in Nirvana is to fall short of the truth concerning that which is unthinkable, unknowable prior to the moment of attainment. Thus questioned, the Buddha was in the position of someone asked to discourse on colour and perspective to an audience consisting of people blind from birth.

Though the Buddhist and Taoist systems of belief and practice differ in some respects, their philosophic base (allowing for differences of terminology) is virtually one and the same. This seems to have been so from a time prior to the two millennia of interaction during which they existed side by side in China. My own explanation of this fact is that Buddhist and Taoist sages, by cultivating inner stillness leading to full intuitive perception of the nature of reality, arrived independently at the same conclusion – a conclusion to which Chinese writers sometimes give the simple name, Not Two. When, to use a Taoist metaphor, wisdom's moon rises in the mind, though different individuals may have their own way of describing its appearance, the moon itself is the same for all.

In hinting at the nature of reality as perceived by yogins far advanced towards Enlightenment, the term 'Not Two' is preferable to the assertion 'All is One', any affirmation being misleading in such a context. 'Not Two' connotes no dualism of creator and created, no ultimate difference in nature between the relative (or perceptible) and absolute (or intangible) aspects of reality. Whatever can be apprehended – a peerless pearl, a discarded shoe, a fragrant rose, a heap of dung, the stupendous cosmos, a single grain of sand, a multitude of objects, a perfect vacuum or void – all alike are manifestations of the infinite, undifferentiated Chên-Ju,[1] the As-It-Is or

[1]Pronounced 'jên-ru'.

That-Which-Is, also called (by Buddhists as well as Taoists) the Tao. This Ultimate or Absolute, if those terms are applicable, does not lie above, behind or beyond its manifestations, for these are Not Two. To use some analogies that are helpful only to a limited extent, pictures projected on a cinema screen have no existence apart from the light of which they are composed; a cloud, now dense and black, now diffused and white, is still the same mass of vapour from which colour and density or the lack of them can by no means be separated, though vapour is vapour whatever these may be. Chên-Ju, being void in the sense of having no intrinsic form or colour, is nevertheless capable of manifesting innumerable forms, colours, degrees of density, etc., etc., etc., none of which can exist apart from it for a single moment. Chên-Ju equates with the Tao in its 'mother' aspect (formless); its manifestations equate with the 'child' aspect (having form). These are Not Two.

In some ways, the sea and its waves provide a good analogy. Waves can be distinguished by size, colour and relative distance from the observer, who is nevertheless aware that these seemingly approaching blue, green and white entities have no identity apart from the colourless watery waste whose uniform composition they share. Were one to conceive of a God or of an Absolute apart from and in any sense other than the totality of the universe, that would be to demean His (its) majesty; for whatever is apart from something else or other than something else cannot be infinite, since infinity precludes otherness. Chên-Ju transcends personal and impersonal, creator and created, just as it transcends all other dualisms.

(b) THE APPLICATION OF THIS TEACHING

To have at least a general concept of this truth, preferably based on some degree of intuitive perception of its validity, is the starting-point for every kind of advanced yoga, for the very word yoga connotes joining – the merging of the individual in the whole, whether by *achieving* union (as some mystics suppose) or by *realising* an identity that has existed from the first, although thickly veiled from sight by the ego-centred delusion of individual existence. A merely intellectual concept, however, cannot lead beyond the starting-point; it is useful only in revealing the direction that yogic practice must take. Beyond that, it is a matter of actually experiencing the truth of being, of transforming a piece of knowledge gleaned perhaps from books into something 'felt in the bones' that gradually (or suddenly) becomes as

real to the yogin as the heat of fire or coldness of ice. Mere knowledge
has to be replaced, then, by the direct fruit of experience; it is this
towards which yogic practice tends.

Everyone who has grasped the essential meaning of Not Two
recognises that appearances can be grossly deceptive. What once
seemed deep may well prove to be a shallow wordy confusion. What
once seemed simple to the point of being elementary may have
implications or consequences so profound as to extend beyond all
levels of consciousness to the very root of being. Or, again, it may
actually be quite elementary at one level of application, yet exceedingly profound at another. This is true of many of the exercises in this
book; those suited to the veriest beginnners sometimes continue to be
employed by adepts already approaching the final stages of the Way.
From the Tibetan lama, Dudjom Rinpoche, who is one of the great
yoga teachers of our time, I learned that an adept, on mastering the
highest class of practices, is advised not to relinquish those at other
levels, but to alternate high and low. Thus even such a simple
meditative exercise as counting the inhalations and exhalations of the
breath may be continued by some adepts right up to the point, just
short of Enlightenment, at which all practices are finally abandoned in
favour of pure contemplation. Though there is not one practice set
forth in this book that goes beyond the category termed simple, that
does not mean that their results cannot be profound. Where they have
been specially simplified for use by Western newcomers to the Way,
no change has occurred in their essence.

Westerners drawn to Buddhism by their admiration for the
emphasis it places on self-endeavour (as opposed to the stress placed
by theists on supernatural aid) are sometimes inclined to dismiss all
rituals (including bowing, chanting, making offerings, etc.) as super-
stitious mumbo-jumbo. This, however, is an error. In the East, there
is no Buddhist sect which dispenses with them; even Zen followers
and Theravadins, who well recognise the dangers of rituals, practice
them daily. Bowing, ceremoniously burning incense and so on
become empty nonsense only if it is supposed that any heavenly
beings are pleased thereby; all rituals are absurd if (as was the case
with certain Brahmins in the Buddha's time) they are performed with
the expectation that correct performance will automatically bring
about desired results. It was this misconception that the Buddha had
in mind when he listed ritualism as one of the dangers to correct
understanding and therefore to progress along the Way. On the other
hand, rituals employed for their psychological effects upon those who
perform them are universally esteemed by Buddhists (barring a few

Western converts led astray by misunderstandings of Zen or Theravada texts, or else by their own revulsion against the ritualism of the churches to which they or their fathers formerly belonged). In prostrating himself before a statue of the Buddha, offering incense and flowers, etc., the Buddhist adept does not seek to please the Buddha, but to express (and cultivate within himself) reverence and awe for what he conceives to be the highest and noblest wisdom accessible to mankind. The Mahayana school of Buddhism has gone further than this by devising techniques in which body, speech and mind are all employed in activities which have exceedingly beneficial psychological effects upon those instructed in their proper use.

Buddhism is full of paradox. For example, though no notion of a creator is entertained, great stress is laid upon the need for faith and piety. By faith is meant not trust in a benevolent deity avid for love, praise and obedience, but conviction that, beyond the seeming reality misreported by our senses which is inherently unsatisfactory, lies a mystery which, when intuitively perceived, will give our lives undreamed-of meaning and endow the most insignificant objects with holiness and beauty. (It should be understood that the term 'beyond' used in this context is strictly speaking incorrect, being used only figuratively for the intangible aspect of the Not Two.) By piety is meant profound respect for the sources of this wisdom, namely the Buddha, the Teaching and the Community (of Buddhas, Bodhisatt-vas, monks, nuns and laymen who have penetrated, or are now engaged upon penetrating, to its core). Piety is expressed not merely by making prostrations and offering incense and flowers, though these actions have their value in instilling reverence and awe into the mind, but chiefly by shunning whatever does not tend to the true welfare and happiness of sentient beings, by zealously practising whatever does tend towards those ends, by esteeming and assisting one's '*dharma*-friends' (teachers and fellow adepts) and by ceaselessly seeking to promote the weal and happiness of all. 'All' naturally includes not just beings but also the environment which (as the doctrine of Not Two makes abundantly clear) is most intimately connected with them, there being no such thing as apartness either within or without the entire cosmic realm.

The need for piety in the sense of feeling the utmost respect for what lies 'above' and 'beyond' the narrow confines of oneself (as ordinarily understood) is one of the reasons why I believe in preserv-ing at least some of the traditional externals that have, since very ancient times, gone hand in hand with yogic practice in the East. That those traditions have been retained for centuries is just because they

have been found helpful in promoting attitudes and states of mind
conducive to progress with the essential practices. In this matter, I
tend to be conservative, but I acknowledge the right of adepts in the
modern West to choose how far to go in maintaining or discarding the
'frills' of traditional practice, while enjoining on them that their
decision should never result from carelessness or idleness; it should be
made for reasons closely connected with the need to progress swiftly
and surely along the Way.

(c) NO DOGMAS

Buddhism is the least dogmatic of religions (although Taoism bids fair
to equal it in this respect). There is not one doctrine to which a
Buddhist must subscribe on pain of being dismissed from the fold.
The Buddha, having undergone the supreme consciousness-
transforming experience that led to his becoming an Enlightened
One, at first decided not to preach what he deemed to be a doctrine
beyond the comprehension of the unenlightened; but, moved by the
sufferings of sentient beings, he subsequently consented to expound
the Way to the extent that it can be encompassed in words. Far from
claiming divine inspiration, he exhorted his disciples to take nothing
on trust, but to put his teachings to the test of experience, to accept
them only if they were found to work and to accord with the intuitions
that would come to them as they progressed with their practice. Thus
Buddhism is a mystical doctrine, being the fruit of direct intuitive
perception and by no means grounded on a divinely inspired set of
scriptures. The Buddha's oral teachings were memorised and transmitted from teacher to disciple for several generations before being
committed to writing, so there was room for divergences of interpretation to creep in. Today, there are some who hold that they are best
represented by the Pali-language version subscribed to by the
Theravadin Buddhists of South-east Asia; whereas others hold to the
Chinese and Tibetan translations of the Mahayana version originally
written in the Sanskrit language that were followed in China and Tibet
before the coming of the communists and still have many followers in
such countries as Korea and Japan. The divergence between
Theravada and Mahayana is greatest with regard to externals and to
methods of practice, least with regard to doctrine and to the necessity
for self-discipline, contemplation (meditation), wisdom and compassion in following the Way. The yogic practices in Part II of this book
are derived chiefly from Chinese sources; of Tibetan yogas I have been

able to say much less, as the majority are confined to adepts who have been properly initiated by a qualified teacher. Nevertheless, much of what has been said in the present section on the subject of theory derives from what I have learnt from Tibetan as well as Chinese teachers.

For all that there are no dogmas, one would hardly call oneself a Buddhist unless one accepted Enlightenment as a valid intuition of the nature of reality, from which it follows that the Enlightened One's exposition of the Way is correct and that the path to Enlightenment as proclaimed by him is an excellent one to follow. As generally understood, to be a Buddhist means to reverence the Triple Gem, namely the Buddha, the Dharma (meaning the Doctrine he proclaimed) and the Sangha (meaning the Community). This last is often taken to mean the Order of Monks, but in a wider (and, I think, truer) sense it connotes all Buddhas, Bodhisattvas and ordinary people who have successfully trod or are now sincerely treading the Way.

I do not think that one has necessarily to be a Buddhist in order to embark upon the practices described in the following pages, for to put teachings to the test of experience before accepting their validity is to accord with the Buddha's own injunction. Buddhism, though mystical in its origin and its goal, that is to say based on direct intuition transcending ordinary states of consciousness, is nevertheless firmly grounded in common sense, on a realistic perception of the unsatisfactoriness of life for those unable to see beyond the realm of data presented by our senses. Its contemplative practices tend towards a heightening and expansion of consciousness; being wholesome, they can lead only to the welfare of the adept and those around him – never to their woe, unless very improperly applied. Even so, being a Buddhist myself, I cannot help supposing that a study of Buddhist works and an inclination to accept their teaching will assist the adept on his Way.

2

Some Mahayana Buddhist Concepts

(a) FORM AND VOID

'Form' here connotes all that pertains to the tangible aspect of reality, including every phenomenon that can be apprehended by the senses and therefore has the appearance of being an individual entity, such as a tree or a bird, a leaf or a feather, or the tip of one of the 'hairs' composing a feather. 'Void' is not to be understood in the sense of mere nothingness, but of no-*thing*-ness. It connotes the intangible aspect of reality – an immeasurable ocean of being or consciousness, formless, colourless, without attributes or qualities of any kind whatsoever; an undifferentiated unity stretching from infinity to infinity and present everywhere. It is the non-substance of which the entire universe is composed. Form and void are Not Two!

Yogic adepts are taught never to lose sight of the intrinsic voidness of phenomena. This might lead one to suppose that phenomena possessing colour, shape, form, density, etc., are unreal like a dream, a mirage, a vision; indeed they *are* unreal, if by unreality is meant that they are void of own-self, of egohood, being merely transitory, ever-changing, interdependent manifestations of the void; nevertheless, they are altogether *real* for the very reason that they share the nature of the void, which alone is eternal, non-dependent, self-existing. Seemingly dream-like phenomena and the intensely real void are Not Two.

This is a matter of immense consequence to yogic adepts. From the very beginning they should strive to understand the non-dual nature of reality. In meditation, the mind seeks to leap beyond the realm of form and come face to face with the self-existent void; this is important not only for the purposes of meditation, but also in learning to accept with equanimity both loss and gain and all the ups and downs of life in the sure knowledge that, in an ultimate sense, nothing *can* be lost or gained, or rise or fall, or progress or retrogress as, except in the realm of mere appearances, everyone and everything is forever complete. With the dawning of Enlightenment when the Way has been followed to the end, there will come full comprehension of Not Two, a perfect reconciliation of form and void, for the last vestiges of dualistic thought will have been transcended. This teaching is the basis of the doctrine set forth in the next section.

(b) THE ONE MIND OR PURE CONSCIOUSNESS

The various Buddhist sects use differing terminology for what all accept as universal truths. Thus , when Ch'an (Zen) followers speak of the One Mind and Wei Shih followers speak of Pure Consciousness (literally Consciousness Only), they are both pointing to a truth that advanced physicists are already beginning to apprehend, namely that 'the stuff of the universe is mind-stuff', to quote Sir James Jeans, who tentatively put forward this notion towards the beginning of this century. In other words, matter reduced to its ultimate constituent proves to be not matter detectable by scientific means, but a 'stuff' (or 'non-stuff') closely analogous to, and probably identical with, mind or consciousness, whichever one may choose to call it. Yogic adepts who have reached states of consciousness transcending dualistic perception have long been unanimous in affirming this truth, which negates all distinction between spirit and matter, mind and matter, animate and inanimate, except as convenient terms to use when talking at the level of dualism and relativity, that is to say the level perceived during everyday states of consciousness. Still more important, since mind has no dimensions, your mind, my mind and Mind Itself are found to be essentially a unity. This explains what is meant by saying that the Buddha, upon Enlightenment, attained to all-knowledge; when illustory divisions have vanished, minds are found to be Mind coextensive with the whole of reality and thus all-embracing. Going even further, it is set forth in the Hua Yen (Avatamsaka) Sutra that, on this account, it is sentient beings themselves who are, collectively, the creators of all that comes to pass throughout the universe. This last is a doctrine so difficult to understand, prior to the attainment of penetrating intuitive wisdom, that we need scarcely be concerned with it here except that, by demonstrating that there are no bounds whatever to what sentient beings can individually or collectively do, it helps to explain why advanced yogins sometimes develop seemingly magical powers, such as telepathy, clairvoyance, levitation, kinemorphosis, etc., as by-products of their practice. These, however, are held to have only slight intrinsic value and to become a positive hindrance to progress should anyone seek deliberately to develop them or feel elated and puffed up at the thought of being able to use them; for then their possession leads to increase instead of diminuition of the arch-foe of successful yogic practice, namely the illusory ego.

Proper understanding of the One Mind or Pure Consciousness doctrine leads to realisation that 'Mind is the King', that true yogic progress pertains to mind alone, body and speech being no more than mind's adjuncts. Such realisation makes it easier to comprehend the doctrine of *karma* set forth below.

(c) *KARMA* AND REBIRTH

Buddhists do not accept the view that life begins with conception and ends with death followed either by life everlasting or by extinction. Throughout each current lifespan, a person sets in motion, by his activities of body, speech and mind, an accumulation of very powerful forces. These, added to what remains of similar accumulations made in former lives, condition his development during the present life-span; and, added to the accumulations that will occur in future lives, will condition a long sequence of rebirths to which there can be no end until Enlightenment, by lifting him above dualistic thought and all the ego-delusions that spring therefrom, sets him free forever from the wheel of life and death, whereafter there is no hindrance to his passing forever into Nirvana. These action-generated forces are known as *karma* and it is this which fully explains the inequalities of life. Good *karma*, resulting from the paring away of ego-centred thoughts, words and actions, leads to progress towards Enlighten-ment; bad *karma*, resulting from thoughts, words and actions tending towards the intensification of egocentricity, leads to retrogression along the Way; both govern the circumstances into which we are reborn. From the delusion of egohood arise the three fires of evil, namely inordinate desire/aversion, passion and delusion. (In some Buddhist texts, one comes upon references to heavens and hells, these being the names given to transient states of happiness and misery that result respectively from good and evil *karma*. Heavens and hells are not interpreted literally, except sometimes at the popular level of understanding; and even those Buddhists who do suppose them to be actual places on a spiritual plane recognise that they have nothing to do with a system of rewards and punishments arbitrarily imposed by a pleased or outraged deity, for undergoing them is seen to be the fruit of one's own actions of body, speech and mind that will endure only until the karmic forces that gave rise to it become exhausted; whereafter other states of birth and rebirth will be entered upon.)

The yogic adept, by persistently reducing his inordinate desires (and their converse, aversions), passions and delusions, liberates his mind from all that gives rise to evil *karma* and, instead, creates good *karma*, that is to say *karma* free from the outflows that keep him bound to the wheel of life and death. The higher yogas especially are short cuts to liberation and consequent Enlightenment.

A basic guide to good action free from outflows was presented by the Buddha in the form of what are called the Four Noble Truths. These are: (i) Life is inseparable from suffering (a broad term used to cover not only mental and physical pain, but also boredom, frustration, disappointment, bereavement, loss, illness, old age, death and all unsatisfactory states whether mild or severe); (ii) suffering has a cause – inordinate desire/aversion; (iii) suffering can be alleviated by cessation of inordinate desire/aversion (on which passions and delusions, too, are contingent); and (iv) its cessation is achieved by right views, right intention, right speech, right conduct, right livelihood, right endeavour, right mindfulness and right meditation. These, giving rise to healthy states of body, speech and mind, will generate good *karma* and lead swiftly towards Enlightenment.

(d) EGOLESSNESS

It is not held that sentient beings have anything in the nature of a soul that passes unchanging from life to life. Indeed, since all phenomena are found to be void of own-being, man cannot be said to possess any sort of ego-entity; that so many people are propelled through life chiefly by desires for egoistic gratification is due to their deludedly clinging to the conviction that 'I' is apart from 'other'. In reality, what is commonly taken to be a person existing in his own right is no more than a wave-like succession of transformations taking place in the Not Two. (It has to be admitted that ego-delusion is immensely strong in most people, and that one needs to be a sage of sages in order to overcome it altogether – yet this certainly can be done, and is in fact what yoga is all about.) What passes from lifespan to lifespan is more nearly analogous to a wave than to a static soul or being; for waves, while retaining their seeming identity as they move forward, are actually discarding and replacing the water of which they are composed so swiftly that a wave that breaks on the shore has nothing but its form in common with that same wave when viewed while still a couple of hundred yards away. The form remains to the end; the composition changes continuously. The same is true of an 'individual', both physically and mentally, within a single lifespan, let alone over many lives. A man of twenty-eight can often be recognised by people who last saw him at the age of seven or fourteen, yet every particle of his body (and of his mental components) will have changed several times since then. To the extent that the boy of seven and the old man of seventy are or are not the same person, so are a man in this current lifespan and the next the same or not the same. What is commonly mistaken for a soul or for an ego-entity is rather a continuum composed of a host of ever-changing and yet coherent tendencies, idiosyncrasies, habits of mind and so on. As the changes are orderly and seldom abrupt, a recognisable 'individuality' passes from one life to the next and to the next and the next, becoming ever less recognisable as the decades and centuries go by. The sum of a person's mental-emotional components at the time of death will presumably be much the same as the sum with which he is reborn, assuming that he does not linger very long in the intermediate state between death and rebirth (called in Tibetan the *bardo*).

Meditation on the absence of a permanent ego is very important to a yogic adept. It helps him to overcome egocentric desires and aversions that are, above all else, responsible for the accumulations of *karma* that lead endlessly from lifespan to lifespan until liberation is won. It is especially valuable in assisting the generation of wisdom and compassion – the twin necessities for Enlightenment.

(e) THE BODHISATTVA VOW

Recognition that the illusory ego is a man's chief enemy, the instigator of his follies, cruelties, aggressions and other displeasing characteristics, naturally gives rise to compassion, since this involves gladly doing for others what the egocentric person does gladly only for himself. With the fading of the false distinction between 'I' and 'other' comes loving respect for one's fellow sentient beings and for the environment as a whole. Thus wisdom stimulates compassion. Conversely, compassion stimulates wisdom, for the less egocentric our thoughts and conduct, the more we perceive the identity of 'self' and 'other', which is the beginning of wisdom. By Mahayana Buddhist adepts compassion is so highly esteemed that every new aspirant for liberation is advised, at the very moment of embarking on the Way, to take a vow that runs as follows:

'I vow that when I attain to Enlightenment, I shall renounce the opportunity to enter upon the bliss of final Nirvana and voluntarily undergo rebirth within the cosmos, there to function as a source of assistance and encouragement to other sentient beings until the time comes when not one of them remains piteously wandering through the round of birth and death. However many aeons it may take for all of them to be ready to enter upon final bliss, I shall not enter before them, for who knows how many of them have been my mothers or otherwise dear to me in former lives?'

It is believed that Bodhisattvas (literally Enlightenment Beings) have the power to appear in whatever forms are best suited to their task – human, animal, divine, demonic, etc. Thus the Bodhisattva Manjusri was said to appear to pilgrims on sacred Mount Wu T'ai, sometimes as a monk, sometimes as a beggar or as a fellow pilgrim, according to need.

(f) THE CELESTIAL BUDDHAS AND BODHISATTVAS

Western people, seeing these beings represented iconographically, are apt to take them for deities, which they are not. They are Enlightened Ones (Buddhas) or Enlightenment Beings (Bodhisattvas) – the distinction is never very clear – who, in pursuance of the vow just mentioned, spend aeon upon aeon instructing, encouraging and assisting unenlightened sentient beings, in this world and all others, there being as many worlds in all as there are grains of sand in the Ganges river. Another explanation given to account for the existence of these beings is that they are embodiments or personifications of certain abstract qualities inherent in the One Mind and therefore in the minds of all, such as Wisdom (Manjusri Bodhisattva), Compassion (Avalokitesvara Bodhisattva), Right Activity (Samandabhadra Bodhisattva), etc., etc. Viewed in this light, they are often made the focus of particular types of meditation, such as the healing yogas described later in Part II of this book. These healing yogas are centred on the figure of Kuan Yin (also known as Kuan Shih Yin in Chinese, Kwannon in Japanese), a female embodiment of the energy of compassion, often depicted in male form under the Sanskrit name Avalokitesvara or Avalokita, and the Tibetan name Chenresigs. A common English name for her, 'the Chinese Goddess of Compassion',

Gateway to Wisdom

is, of course, a misnomer based on a misunderstanding of her nature. Whether Kuan Yin is chiefly thought of as an Enlightenment Being who labours for others in pursuance of her vow, or whether the Western adept prefers to think of her as an embodiment of the energy of compassion, personified for yogic purposes, does not matter, for it will be found that meditations and yogic healing practices focused on her are extraordinarily effective, no matter in what light one regards this being. The same is broadly true of several other Celestial Buddhas and Bodhisattvas, who may be regarded either as actual beings or as embodiments of qualities and energies for psychological purposes.

(g) SELF-POWER AND OTHER-POWER

Buddhism is notable among the world's religions for its emphasis on self-endeavour (as opposed to reliance on divine aid) as the sole means to liberation. However, the Buddha, being opposed to the dogmatism displayed by a great many of the world's religious leaders, believed in the value of *upaya* (skilful means). People with different mental endowments, different characteristics, or at different levels of attainment, have all to be catered for. Therefore ways have been found for all of them, including those with little confidence in their own powers and/or with a natural inclination towards devotional practices. Among these ways is taking recourse to other-power, which seems to be in direct contradiction to the more usual Buddhist practice; that it is not so will be apparent once the relation of self-power to other-power is properly understood, for in reality they are the same. Here we shall take other-power as related to the Bodhisattva Kuan Yin as our example. It is recorded that this Bodhisattva, by the power of her compassionate vow not to enter the bliss of final Nirvana unless all beings were able to enter, created a Pure Land known as the Potala, into which errant beings can enter freely merely by fervently desiring to be reborn there under conditions ideally favourable for treading the rest of the Way leading to liberation and Nirvana. Those who believe in and choose this means of treading the Way may be said to resort to other-power, namely the compassionate power of Kuan Yin Bodhisattva.

What, in effect, is the difference between the self-power and other-power methods? It will be found to be wholly a matter of conceptualisation. I may rely upon self-power to overcome the three fires of evil by developing boundless compassion, emancipating myself from the grasp of ego-delusion, and seeking immersion in the undifferentiated non-substance of the cosmos – pure consciousness. Another person may rely upon the power of Kuan Yin to overcome the three fires of evil by drawing upon the energy of boundless compassion latent in Mind, but now embodied for yogic purposes in the lovely form of Kuan Yin, in order to be liberated from ego-delusion and enter her Pure Land. Now, compassion is compassion, an energy latent in my mind, your mind and in Mind Itself. Whether I conceive of it as being internal or external to myself will make no difference, provided that I develop it to the full. I can picture it as welling up from within my heart, or as being directed towards me by the Bodhisattva Kuan Yin; in either case, it will prove an admirable antidote to egocentricity and loosen the grasp of ego-delusion. Again, I may seek to immerse myself in the non-substance of the cosmos, or else to enter Kuan Yin's Pure Land, but the point is that Kuan Yin's Pure Land is no other than the undifferentiated ocean of pure consciousness that becomes apparent to the adept when all ego-born desire and aversion have been swept away. These are two names for the same no-*thing*! Two men journeying to Tibet for the first time in their lives may conceive of it very differently until they come to see it for themselves. When that happens, it will be the same place for both of them. Mind and its latent energies, including that of compassion, are not spatial entities with an entrance and exit, a beginning and an end. In that context, to speak of inside and outside, internal and external, self-power and other-power is to make meaningless distinctions. Mind is everywhere – inside and outside, there being no difference between them.

Whether or not the matter thus stated will satisfy logicians, I do not know; but it is interesting to note that Dr Daisets Suzuki, who spent a great part of his life introducing Zen to the West, wrote a final book before he died, entitled *Shin: Japan's Greatest Gift to the West* – Shin being the Japanese name for Pure Land practice. In Eastern countries, there has rarely been any doubt that the self-power and other-power methods of attainment are identical in their results, though set forth in widely different conceptual terms.

(h) SUPERNATURAL BEINGS

What is said under this head is just by the way and merely for clarification, the existence of supernatural beings such as gods and demons having no direct bearing on yogic progress, except that demons (alias negative psychological factors) do trouble most meditators. Gods

and goddesses should not be confused with the special category of
Celestial Buddhas and Bodhisattvas described above.

Like the Buddha himself, Buddhists accept the existence of various
orders of supernatural beings, but set no store by them in the context
of cultivating the Way. Wherever Buddhism spread in Asia, instead of
attempting to suppress the indigenous religions, it incorporated local
beliefs together with the existing iconography, and in many cases
transmuted those beliefs into psychological instruments for use in
cultivating the Way. Gods and demons, though accepted into the fold
(and not infrequently *converted* (!) to become temple guardians and so
forth), are held to be part of the natural order like animals or fish and
therefore subject to nature's immutable laws – to birth, growth, decay
and death in accordance with the time-scale proper to each species. To
what extent they are regarded as actual beings like those depicted in
paintings and statues, or as psychological influences either benign or
malignant, varies from one person to another, but rarely are they
accorded much importance by followers of the Way, unless in the
capacity of guardians with functions not very different from those of
gatekeepers (gods), or as sources of hindrance to meditation
(demons).

In Tibet, especially, where the iconographic range of gods and
demons is enormous, these beings – or their likenesses – have been
utilised psychologically. Meditators are taught to recognise the entire
pantheon of gods and demons and even of Celestial Buddhas and
Bodhisattvas as emanations of their own minds, or as embodiments of
positive and negative psychological factors. In China, there has
traditionally been a tendency to treat supernatural beings, other than
Buddhas and Bodhisattvas, with circumspection, to be scrupulously
polite when compelled to have dealings with them, but to remain at a
respectful distance whenever possible. An exception is made of
wandering ghosts, those of dead people who, for one reason or
another, are earth-bound for a time. In Chinese Buddhist monasteries, the monks never started a meal without first making offerings
of rice to those unhappy creatures; and, in connexion with rites for the
dead, the wandering ghosts used to be feasted ceremoniously at the
expense of the bereaved, this being deemed a way of making merit on
behalf of the departed. I warmly admired this compassionate attitude;
if the wandering ghosts were really there, they must have been deeply
grateful for such kind attentions; if they were not there, no harm was
done and considerable good achieved by making living human beings
conscious of the need to extend compassion to every kind of creature,
visible or invisible.

According to Mahayana Buddhist tradition, the universe is peopled
by six main orders of being – gods, titans (jealous of the gods),
humans, animals, *pretas* (hungry ghosts) and denizens of hell (demons
and their victims, of whom the latter are held to be only transients who
will undergo happier rebirths once their evil *karma* has been
expiated).

3

Attitude

A very important adjunct to yogic practice is maintaining at all times a suitable attitude of mind. Buddhist adepts, generally happy in themselves, as they are content with simple things and joyful at the thought of the path to liberation lying before them, are taught to feel immense concern for the hosts of sentient beings who wander blindly from birth to birth performing actions that tend towards heavy accumulations of *karma*. The search for liberating wisdom has always to be accompanied by the cultivation of unlimited compassion for all in need of it, whether humans, animals or ghosts. An important aim for all adepts is the generation of *bodhi citta* (meaning an Enlightened mind – or heart). This requires abstention from every kind of deliberate hurt to others – murder and theft of course, but also feelings or words of anger, hatred, envy, malice and so on. Unkindly gossip and wounding speech have also to be shunned, together with lying and every sort of dishonesty. It goes without saying that a dedicated adept would not think of deliberately taking the life of any sentient creature down to the smallest insect (mosquitoes included) or most repulsive reptile. I know of a small hermitage in India which was abandoned by the Tibetan nuns who lived there because, in winter when they were cut off by snow, the rats used to eat up most of their scanty stocks of grain; it never entered their minds that a more convenient solution would be to kill off the rats; they would have been appalled had anyone suggested it.

Avoidance of deliberate hurt to others is only the negative aspect of the morality enjoined upon cultivators of the Way. The positive aspect requires the generous bestowal of all the kindness, comfort, help and support of which one is capable. Liberation is the result of diminishing egocentricity until not a shred of it remains; the prime antidote to egocentricity is compassion.

The whole of Buddhist morality can be summed up in two sayings, the first of which is: 'Treat every being without exception as though it has been your mother in a previous life!' This injunction, taken in the context of the aeon upon aeon of lives we have lived already, is by no means exaggerated or fanciful. The second is seemingly of the same kind, but much more profound, as it has meanings at many levels that correspond closely to the nature of reality; it runs: 'See all beings as Buddhas! Hear all sounds as Mantra! Behold all places as Nirvana!' These were the very words of the teaching I received when I first set out upon the Way.

See all beings as Buddhas! Potentially all beings *are* Buddhas, for it is taught that every single one of them will attain to Enlightenment eventually. In another sense, all beings are already Buddhas, for all alike share the Buddha Nature, which is another term for the Not Two nature of reality of which everyone partakes. Whereas it is humanly impossible to obey the injunction 'Love thy neighbour as thyself', since some people and animals attract us from the very moment we set eyes upon them, while others repel us deeply (until we are far advanced along the Way), it is entirely possible to treat even the most revolting beings with compassion – which involves being able and willing to sympathise with them. Obviously whatever characteristics make a person thoroughly unlikeable are afflictions no less deserving of compassion than blindness or an incurable malady. Nobody can enjoy being universally disliked; recognising this, it becomes easy to bear with such a person, to be kind and feel no resentment towards him. It is even easier when we reflect, in all sincerity, that we are actually standing in the presence of one destined to become an Enlightened One – a Buddha. To show respect and kindness, even where we can as yet feel not the least inclination to love, is a very rewarding attitude, too, for it is likely to win us friends and enable us to avoid making any enemies at all. This part of the triple injunction, then, is by far the easiest of the three to put into immediate practice.

Hear all sounds as Mantra! This, on the contrary, is exceedingly difficult to practise in this age of blaring transistor radios, pneumatic road-drills, sixteen-wheel trucks, cranes, fork-lifts and other sources of ear-splitting noise on every hand. 'The companionable roar of the cliff-dwelling tiger', to quote a Taoist poem mentioned in Part I of this book, would sound sweet indeed compared with the horrid cacophony of a modern metropolis. All the same, there are ways of dealing with this problem, although it can hardly have been foreseen by those who framed the injunction many centuries ago when even man-made sounds were close to those of nature, such as the creaking of wooden wheels or the jingle of harness. My Chinese and Tibetan teachers, being barely acquainted with the noises made by machines, other than the occasional roar and rattle of a passing country bus or four-wheel truck, had no difficulty in preserving the ancient belief that the totality of sound in the universe is mantric sound, a term probably synonymous with 'the music of the spheres'. Doubtless they were right and doubtless the belief is still true today, for the most unnatural sounds conceivable are man-made, and what is man or what are the tools he uses but products of nature at one or more removes? Dealing with the problem, then, entails first acceptance of the notion that desire and aversion proceed from our own minds, hence beauty and discord relate not to real things but to our own deluded perception of That-Which-Is. It is we ourselves who make such deluded pronouncements as that this or that sound is beautiful, this or that sound ugly. Neither ugliness nor beauty are relevant to the nature of That-Which-Is – Chên-Ju. Knowing this, we can learn to transmute a discordant din, as it seems to us, into melodious sounds. By a strong effort of will that seems to lead us into the realm of make-believe, though actually it springs from perception of the subtle nature of reality, we can hear the thump of machinery as the rhythmic beating of a ceremonial drum, or the roar of traffic as the howling of wind screaming through caves at a high altitude or as the sound of the ocean hurling itself against a rocky coast. This is not make-believe, but an indication of our success in the conquest of false distinctions. Nothing lies outside the Way, and what is the fearsome caterwauling of a great metropolis such as London, Tokyo or Los Angeles in comparison with the music and silence of the spheres? Each adept must, in his own way, transmute discord into beauty by the power of his own imagination. That it can be done, I know from experience; for many years ago I learned to transmute the chugging and screeching of trishaws being driven in bottom gear round and round a piece of grass outside the windows of my meditation room into the rattle of lamas' drums and the booming of two rivers rushing together at the base of a hill in Sikkim known as Tashiding. Truly a degree of effort is involved, but it is effort well worth making.

Behold all places as Nirvana! This is entirely logical, for there is absolutely nowhere that is not a manifestation of the sublime reality that will be perceived in its fullness with the dawning of Enlightenment. What we take to be winsome beauty or repulsive ugliness arise from within ourselves, being the fruits of false perception stemming from dualistic thought. Not a single cranny of the universe differs in nature from the sublime reality of the Chên-Ju, the Tao! Dealing with ugliness as reported by the eye is simple in comparison with rising above the discord that assaults our ears, for the illusory nature of visual ugliness or beauty is more obvious. As recorded in more than one of my earlier books, I was once quite overwhelmed by the beauty of what I took to be a mass of scarlet blossom, until I drove close enough to discern that the illusion was created by some trees rising from behind a corrugated iron fence painted over with red lead! For as long as I saw the sight as beautiful, it was movingly beautiful. What changed was not the sight itself, but my concept of its nature. Certainly all places are Nirvana; that it does not lie apart from Here and Now becomes apparent to Enlightened perception. What is needed is not a change of circumstance, but a revolution of mind.

The attitude of a yogic adept to his surroundings must be one of supreme reverence for What Is. Desire and aversion cannot be overthrown in a day – perhaps not in a lifetime – but they must be rigorously subdued until they cease to constitute a grave hindrance to cultivation of the Way. If someone still at the outset of the path makes up his mind to cultivate wisdom and compassion – pursuing the former through reading, learning orally, observation and meditation, and developing the latter by reflecting that his own longings for happiness and well-being are shared by all sentient creatures – his progress is likely to be swift. Even so, he must be wary of entertaining more than a modest satisfaction in the results accomplished. Spiritual pride and the elation caused by notable progresss inflate the ego and thereby send the adept tumbling back to square one on life's snakes and ladders board. One who declares himself to be Enlightened is very sure to be either a charlatan or a person cruelly deluded; for, the closer sages draw to liberation, the more unassuming they become. True sages would pass altogether unnoticed by the world, were it not that, driven by compassion for the welfare of sentient beings, they respond unstintingly to those who desire and are genuinely in need of their guidance.

B PRACTICE

1

Mode of Living and Preparation

(a) RIGHT LIVELIHOOD

Traditionally, Buddhist yogic adepts have tended to be either monks and nuns or cave-dwelling hermits dissevered from worldly ties and thus able to concentrate night and day on their spiritual development; yet there have always been a fair number of laymen who have succeeded in combining the life of ordinary house-holders, involving family responsibilities, with the demands of yogic cultivation and of whole-hearted dedication to that task. This last is the pattern most likely to be followed in the West. To be freed from the burdens of earning a living and supporting parents, spouse or children is certainly a great blessing, but present-day conditions make this an unattainable ideal for a great many people; besides, the loneliness that threatens strict celibates and hermits may lead to frustrations and aberrations more harmful to swift progress than the cares and responsibilities inherent in having a lover or a wife and perhaps several children. The one circumstance of this sort that is totally inimical to yogic progress is wrong liveli-hood. Any profession, any activity that involves knowing hurt to other sentient beings must be ruled out completely. That a butcher, a fisherman, a hunter or a gangster is unqualified to set out upon the yogic path goes without saying; moreover, right livelihood is not easy to equate with the profession of soldier (who must take life when so commanded) or with any form of business activity that involves sharp practice or the gathering of undue pro-fits at the expense of other people. It is really not difficult to draw the dividing line, for everyone must surely be aware of whether or not his manner of earning a living harms other sentient beings or not. Teaching, medicine, nursing are, to all appearance, excellent professions, but not if the work is undertaken in a slipshod manner, or with an eye to emoluments and comfort rather than to the weal and happiness of those served. A teacher must not mislead his pupils by slipshod teaching or defraud them by giving of less than his best – and so on. These are not dogmatic rules, but arise from the nature of the yogic quest.

(b) DIET

Many Buddhists, monks and nuns especially, follow strict dietary rules, but these vary with climate and cultural environment. Chinese monks are strict vegetarians; Tibetan and Mongolian lamas, living as they do where greenery is sparse, are not, though they never willingly take life or have animals specially killed for them. In Southeast Asia, the Theravadin monks sally forth at dawn to receive food offerings from the faithful, none of which may be rejected, whether vegetarian or not. Other Buddhist countries have other customs. There are no hard and fast rules that apply to all, so Western Buddhists have a variety of precedents to follow. What is of the utmost consequence is not to be involved in the deliberate destruction of life; next to that comes the need for abstemiousness, as overeating and greed are both inimical to meditative progress. All self-indulgence is harmful; but so, on the other hand, is an unwise degree of asceticism. Following the middle path between indulgence and unnecessary deprivation is best.

(c) SEX

Unless one has taken monastic vows or embarked upon one of those high yogas that demand every atom of one's energy, there is no need to be celibate, especially as rigid abstention may lead to suppressed longings and tortured fantasies that seriously undermine mental health. Nevertheless, yogic practice does demand avoidance of excess in all things. Mental and physical energies being closely linked, the latter must not be too freely expended to the detriment of the former. Buddhist laymen are free to indulge in sexual intercourse, provided it is not practised to excess and that it does not involve a 'wrong person', which means someone to whom suffering would be caused as a result, or someone whose participation would cause suffering to a third party, say, a wronged spouse or, in the case of a very young girl, parents who would grieve.

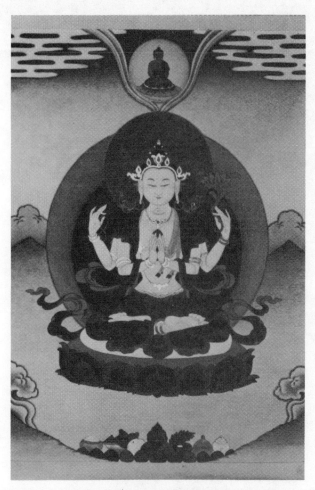

Four-armed Avalokitesvara

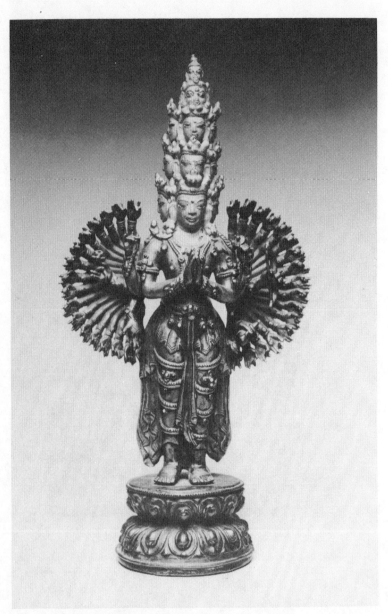

Thousand-armed Avalokitesvara

(d) INTOXICANTS

Buddhists all accept that to imbibe intoxicants, including alcohol, is to transgress one of the five precepts (not to kill, steal, indulge in improper sex, lie or imbibe 'sloth-producing and intoxicating' substances) which serious followers of the Way are expected to abide by for their own sakes, though no one orders them to do so. However, in practice, a fair number of laymen interpret the fifth precept rather liberally, taking it to mean that a limited use of alcohol is acceptable provided that the drinker stops well short of drunkenness, for thus the spirit if not the letter of the law is observed. In all cases, a person serious about yogic practice should drink, if at all, very abstemiously. As to other drugs, such as hashish, opium, heroin, cocaine, LSD, etc., Chinese and Tibetan masters without exception regard their use as harmful to yogic practice and strongly recommend that they be eschewed.

(e) HABITATION

Modern individuals, unless quite wealthy, are seldom free to choose the environment in which they live and work. Obviously beautiful natural surroundings remote from the bustle of cities are ideal for cultivation of the Way; but people precluded by poverty, family obligations or the nature of their employment from seeking such surroundings must learn to adapt their practice to their circumstances, while taking care to sacrifice nothing that is fundamental to their yogic aim. City dwellers can compromise to some extent by spending weekends and annual holidays in places suited to peaceful communion with nature and the attainment of stillness.

Some people, youngsters especially, may be drawn to join one of those communities with members of both sexes and room for children such as one finds at Tassajara in California and which are now springing up in many parts of North America and Europe. Excellent home-grown food, adequate lodging and good teaching are provided in return for labour – in the fields or on community buildings or services, etc. – and the days are programmed so as to allow time for meditation and study. Under circumstances such as these, the work itself takes on a yogic quality. Nevertheless, one should be cautious. It is advisable to know a lot about a community before deciding to join it; and, if at all possible, to stay there for a while so as to make sure of its suitability to one's needs. Above all, no irrevocable commitment should ever be necessary. A community that demands the surrender of personal wealth and property or one that requires a commitment extended far into the future should be avoided; for who is to know what regrets may arise due to incompatibility? There should be no moral, physical or financial restraint on one's leaving (after giving reasonable notice) if and when the time for that arrives.

I visited several communities in the States and Canada to which, were I younger, I should be happy to belong. The members are obviously animated by a spirit of service and by enthusiasm for their work, studies and meditation, besides looking healthy and contented. In such places, there is no atmosphere of false other-worldliness, no attitude of holier than thou, no distressingly emotional air – just quietly joyous involvement in work and meditation reminiscent of the hermitages I used to visit on China's sacred mountains.

Yogic cultivation can, of course, well be undertaken on one's own. With good understanding, one can tread at least the initial stages of the path even where living conditions are deplorable, such as in a prison or a slum, though such conditions do make practice more difficult. So much depends on mental attitude that surroundings are of only secondary importance, which is not quite to say that they are unimportant. The One Mind, the Great Void, the Buddha Nature, the Tao – whatever one may choose to call it – forms the very ground and substance of our being. No person and no place is ever apart from it.

(f)   A BRIEF RÉSUMÉ OF YOGIC AIMS

By no means everyone who makes use of this book is likely to have set his mind on exploring the full extent of the Way; but, for those who do hope to go far along it, I have thought that a brief résumé of aims may be useful here. An aspiring adept seeks: (i) to learn how to eradicate inordinate desires and aversions; (ii) to transmute (not suppress) all negative qualities such as passions and delusions; (iii) to stimulate the flow of intuitive wisdom; (iv) to recognise the holiness of the whole cosmic environment down to the smallest insect or blade of grass; (v) to banish the ego demon and cultivate compassion; and (vii) to take some steps towards that full self-realisation that leads to liberation and Enlightenment.

These tasks involve, from the very outset: (i) awareness and watchfulness over one's actions of body, speech and mind; (ii) the cultivation of inner stillness and of a sense of unity with one's environment; and (iii) the progressive curtailment of ego-centred actions and desires and frequent meditation on the need for ripening compassion – all of these to be accompanied by the unremitting practice of frugality, simplicity, kindness and reverence towards all that is. Increasingly these measures will lead to attaining the inner stillness that confers tranquil joy, freedom from anxiety, fearlessness and, upon occasion, moments of actual bliss. Simultaneously the adept will become ever more happily reconciled to living in the Here and Now and thus go at least a little way towards recognising that Nirvana is not a distant state, but lies all about him, being perceptible to all with eyes to see what lies beneath the realm of mere appearances. Such are the early stages of the path that leads to the giving and enjoyment of happiness in this life.

2

The Bodhi-Mandala and Basic Techniques

(a) INTRODUCTORY

Set forth in this section are the requirements for some of the simpler forms of yogic cultivation as practised by Buddhists; they are cast in traditional form and include practices that may not appeal to those who wish to experiment with yoga without actually subscribing to the teaching of the Enlightened One. For example, some non-Buddhists may like to attempt Buddhist-style healing within the context of their own religion (or lack of belief), in which case what is said under the headings (b) and (c) below may seem irrelevant. Well, the healing method given here may, for all I know, be susceptible to infinite adaptation; but, having been a Buddhist since childhood, I have not ventured to experiment along those lines, so I cannot say how effective the results would be. My own experience has persuaded me that the more closely one conforms with old and tried practices, the greater the measure of success; yet I do accept the possibility of fruitful adaptation.

(b) THE BODHI-MANDALA (HOUSEHOLD SHRINE)

Purity

According to Chinese tradition, the yogic adept should strive to maintain both ritual purity and actual purity of body, speech and mind, and to extend this to the household shrine. Purity of body, speech and mind connotes inward and outward cleanliness, especially during the time that elapses between waking before dawn and entering the shrine for what should normally be the main practice of the day, as Buddhists share with Taoists a preference for the early hours when cosmic *ch'i* circulates most freely. On waking, the first coherent thought should take the form of a powerful aspiration for the welfare and happiness of all sentient beings, followed by a renewal of the Boddhisattva Vow to strive to benefit them aeon upon aeon at whatever cost to oneself. Rising promptly, one evacuates the bowels, bathes and cleanses the mouth. While engaged in these small tasks, one should keep the mind free from turgid emotions and avoid every kind of mental ugliness in favour of a mood of inner stillness and quiet joy – a mood to be maintained, as far as possible, at all other times of the day and night as well. Purity of the Bodhi-Mandala requires that it be kept spotlessly clean and that it should never be entered without first dismissing turgid thoughts, passion, ill will and all such negative feelings, so that gradually the atmosphere in the neighbourhood of the shrine becomes charged with a radiant and tangible stillness, free from thought pollution.

Time

So long as this rule is kept, the shrine may be entered at any time of day or night – the more time spent there the better – but not for purposes unconnected either with keeping it clean or with cultivation.

Place

Ideally the Bodhi-Mandala should be a small room in the uppermost storey of a dwelling. If this cannot be managed, then a quiet corner of any room will do instead, but people making use of the room as a whole for non-yogic purposes should be deterred from entering that particular corner, which should be kept clean, uncluttered and free from disturbance at all times. If there is no space for a small table on which to place a Buddha image and other objects, a special shelf resting on brackets attached to the wall some five feet above floor-level will serve the purpose. If, on the other hand, a small table or cabinet can be placed against the wall, so as to have a flat surface on which to rest the Buddha image, etc., it should be mounted on a step-like base so that the image is at least as high above the floor as the chest of a person standing erect. This requirement applies also to pictures or scrolls hung on the wall behind, or in lieu of, the statue. To place sacred objects at a lower level or, worse still, on the floor is a form of disrespect highly offensive to traditionally-minded Buddhists. In Buddhist Thailand, such disrespect is actually punishable by law. At first sight, this may seem an extreme point of view, but sacred objects are symbols of high spiritual aspiration; their purpose is to generate in the adept's heart the awe and reverence without which yogic practice can scarcely be successful.

Arrangement

Simplicity should be the keynote. The Bodhi-Mandala's contents should be sparse and beautiful, though not necessarily expensive. To obtain precious objects at a cost that is extravagant in relation to one's means would be to flout the requirement of frugality. In the centre of the table, cabinet or shelf should be a likeness of the Buddha and/or of the Celestial Bodhisattva, such as Kuan Yin, on whom one's regular yogic practice is centred; and, in front of this, there should be a space for flowers, incense-burner, lights, etc. (see *Symbolical Offerings* below).The meditation cushion should be so positioned on the floor that the adept sits with the statue or picture at some distance above the level of his eyes. If the Bodhi-Mandala is used by two or more people simultaneously, the cushions should be positioned to suit the convenience of them all.

Symbolical Offerings

These, too, are chiefly important on account of the state of mind they inculcate. They may consist of a single bowl of pure fresh water, or of two small vases of flowers, or be more elaborate; the total effect should be calculated to produce feelings of awe, veneration and happiness. Incense and lights (a pair of candles or Tibetan butter-lamps filled more conveniently with liquid vegetable oil) are generally found to contribute to this effect. A set of five offerings known as *wu kung*, that was almost universally used in China, consists of an incense-burner tightly packed with ash for planting lighted incense-sticks, flanked by a pair of candlesticks that in turn are flanked by a pair of vases containing fresh flowers; and, upon occasion, one or more bowls of fresh uncut fruit are added. The utensils should be as beautiful as possible and kept spotlessly clean. The offerings should not include wilted flowers or bruised fruits. Empty bowls, vases, etc., should not be left upon the table, but the incense-burner, being filled with ash, stands there permanently.

Incense-sticks are used in odd numbers – usually one, three, five, seven or nine. If the room is small and the atmosphere close, one is best. The sticks, on being lighted with a match, are likely to burst into flame at the tips; the flame should not be blown out, but extinguished by waving one hand sharply so as to cause a momentary current of air. They are planted exactly upright in a burner so tightly packed to the brim with ash that they remain erect; then, as they burn down, their ash will fall on to the expanse of ash below and not soil the table or utensils. Of the varieties of incense now commonly available in the West, I prefer the better kinds of Tibetan or Japanese incense-sticks, as their odour is neither over-sweet nor over-pungent. Candles may be of any colour; however, tradition favours red or yellow. Normally these should be rather small and left to burn right down each time, so, that new ones can be placed for each session. If larger candles are used and, for economy's sake, blown out at the end of a session, the blowing out should be done in the manner just described for extinguishing the flame of newly lighted incense. The breath should not be used for this purpose.

Percussion Instruments

These are often employed by adepts because notes struck on them are sometimes an extraordinary help to achieving, quite suddenly, a disposition to inner stillness or even to 'snapping into' an expanded state of consciousness that might take long to attain by other means. One instrument, sparingly used, is sufficient. It may be a metal bowl struck with a wooden mallet wrapped around with cloth like a gong-stick, a sweet-toned bell, a small gong, a wooden 'fish-drum' (a hollow block of resonant wood struck with a wooden mallet of which the striking end, not wrapped with cloth, resembles a conventionalised lotus bud), a Tibetan instrument consisting of two small cymbal-shaped discs of metal alloy joined by a string and held in such a manner that the rims clash together, or a small hand-drum with metal pellets depending from strings that rain thunderously on its two surfaces when it is twirled rapidly backwards and forwards by movements of the wrist. As a prelude to yogic contemplation, a single note is struck on one of these, or the hand-drum caused to rattle very briefly. A single note also marks the end of a session, or the end of one practice and the beginning of another during the same session. Suitable materials for fashioning home-made substitutes are wood, bronze, various alloys, silver, flat strips of jade or slivers of any resonant stone. Percussion instruments are not by any means essential to practice, but a single, beautiful, lingering note may at times thrill the adept with a sudden intimation of spirit permeating the realm of form. This is a mystery I accept without being at all able to explain it. The more complicated use of percussion instruments during yogic rituals, such as the use of bell and drum by a Tibetan lama, requires special instruction from a teacher. From experience in Taoist hermitages, I have learnt that a short melody on a bamboo flute is another aid to stilling the mind before a session.

Further Observations

Some of the matters mentioned in this section may seem quaint and

out of line with modern ways of thinking, but I have found that all
contribute to attaining the special states of consciousness one seeks in
meditation. Mind, as always, is the King. Thus, for example, a small
bowl of water can be mentally transmuted by the adept into rich
offerings as vast in scale as the universe itself by a simple act of
visualisation accompanied by sincere aspiration, or into lighted
lamps, smouldering incense or whatever may be physically lacking.
Effective yoga depends on understanding the infinite power of mind
and on achieving, sometimes with the help of ritualistic means,
expanded states of consciousness. Though making the kinds of
offerings described and also the prostrations dealt with in the following section may seem anachronistic, they are valuable on account of
their psychological effect; they should not be thought of in the same
terms as worship of anthropomorphic deities, but as ancient rituals
intended to reinforce the attitude of mystery and awe that is needed to
carry the adept far along the Way. Suppose that the universe were in
fact the handiwork of a Creator God, would the author of all the
beauties in the universe really take delight in the odour of incense and
burnt offerings? Of course not. Making such trivial gifts to Him
would be like offering a few pence to a billionaire. Still less does the
Enlightened One, having attained Nirvana, require such things from
his followers. It cannot be emphasised too strongly that the 'subject
before a monarch stance' taken by yogins – especially those who are
still at an early stage of the Way – is a necessary part of yogic practice,
not a means of winning favour from divine beings likely to impose
somewhat arbitrary and whimsical rewards and punishments on
their devotees.

(c) PROSTRATION

Asian Buddhists, in accordance with ancient custom, touch their
heads thrice to the floor on entering or leaving a Bodhi-Mandala or
temple. Yogically, this, too, is of great importance because, in
meditation, there is always a danger of being pleased with progress
made; but a single thought of 'Good! *I* am doing much better now'
sends the adept hurtling back to the starting-point; for, since yogic
meditation is aimed at transcending false distinctions between 'I' and
'other', a mood of self-congratulation undoes the achievements
hitherto gained; indeed, it actually *increases* the hold of ego-delusion.
To counteract this danger, it is good to alternate meditation practice
with obeisance to the Buddha. In a Mahayana context, the word

'Buddha' connotes not only the historical founder of Buddhism, but also the Buddha-Principle – the Buddha-Nature inherent in the minds of all sentient beings. By paying reverence to a statue representing the Buddha-Nature, which is also the void, the One Mind, the adept reminds himself that all his seeming personal achievement is in reality a function of everlasting Being, of which people are transient embodiments possessing no ultimate reality apart from its animating force. In an absolute sense, it is not Mr Wang or Mr Smith who attains Enlightenment, this seeming victory being in fact a manifestation of the Buddha-Nature within him – a priceless possession common to all sentient beings. There being, ultimately, no separation between worshipper and worshipped, paying homage to that-which-is-greater-than-self is an effective way of overcoming such baneful backslidings in understanding as the thought '*I* have gone further than poor Mr Li or that inefficient yogin, Mr Jones'.

Prostrations performed in the Bodhi-Mandala or elsewhere at the beginning and end of each session may take one of several forms. (i) The simplest is to kneel on the floor just behind the meditation cushion and, having first made a gesture of homage by placing the hands palm to palm at forehead level, bend forward three times in succession so that the hands, maintaining that palm-to-palm position, thrice touch the floor with the forehead resting upon the joined thumbs. (ii) Chinese Buddhists, however, think it proper to prostrate themselves thrice from a standing position. Each prostration commences with the body held erect, toes almost touching the edge of the meditation cushion, hands pressed palm to palm at breast level. Next, bending knees and body, the adept extends his right arm and places the hand palm downwards on the cushion. Then, with both knees on the ground, he extends his left arm until the hand comes to rest, palm upwards, a few inches in front of the right hand. Moving the right hand forward over the cushion to join it, with both palms now facing upward so that the little fingers lie against each other, he prepares to cup his forehead, which now comes to rest on the upturned palms. The standing position is regained by reversing these movements, and two more prostrations follow. The feet remain side by side, toes close to the cushion, throughout. To avoid ungainliness, the buttocks must be kept well down when the forehead comes to rest upon the palms. Beginners are liable to spoil the beauty of the whole movement by carelessly allowing their buttocks to remain projecting high into the air. I remember being reprimanded for this while living as a monk in the Hua T'ing Monastery near Kunming, where I received my initial training in monastic decorum. 'The English disciple', cried the monk in charge of training, 'is very pious. Even his bottom has become a pagoda!' With a little practice, the whole series of movements will soon acquire a smooth gracefulness that makes them beautiful to watch, especially when performed in unison by several people; there must be precision, but it should seem effortless, not drill-like. (iii) Tibetans also make their three prostrations from the standing position. With the body held erect, the hands are joined palm to palm above the crown of the head, then brought to the levels of throat and breast in turn, the adept meanwhile mentally aspiring to the purity of body, speech and mind thus symbolised. On completing these preliminary gestures and aspirations within the space of a second or so, he falls swiftly to his knees, the feet remaining close together as before, and extends both arms simultaneously so that the hands come to lie palm-upward on the cushion, with the little fingers touching each other, thus forming a shallow bowl in which to cup the forehead, which is swiftly brought to rest in them. With this type of prostration, there are in all three sets of four movements, each set consisting of three gestures with the joined hands followed by a full prostration. Like their Chinese-style counterparts, they are performed with such smoothness, speed and grace as to seem almost effortless.

Tibetan lamas usually require their pupils to perform 100,000 '*grand* prostrations' as part of the qualifications for receiving instruction in the tantric yogas. A grand prostration starts off with the three gestures of aspiration just described; but, on arriving at the kneeling position, the adept shoots out his arms and body until he lies at full length on the ground, and then pays homage by bringing his palms together, fingers pointing skyward above his prostrate head. This is an admirable yogic exercise involving body, speech and mind, for the mind is concentrated throughout on the need to purify those three faculties, and the tongue recites the mantra OM AH HUM, the syllables of which correspond with the three preliminary gestures of aspiration. Besides demonstrating profound reverence for the greater-than-self Buddha-Nature and providing an antidote to egoistic satisfaction in one's yogic progress, the movements exercise all the muscles of the body and thus provide a remedy for the harmful physical effects of sitting for many hours a day motionless in meditation. Therefore many adepts perform from about twenty to a hundred or more grand prostrations at the beginning or end of each meditation session.

Even with the more ordinary types of prostration, beginners unused to making ceremonious gestures are bound to feel – and look – awkward and clumsy until they have mastered them by practice. To mask their clumsiness and, later on, to add particular grace and dignity to movements that have become second nature, it is helpful to wear a long robe – but not longer than ankle-length, lest it get under the feet while one is rising from a prostration and result in ludicrous efforts to avoid falling down. It is, in any case, very usual for adepts to keep a long robe made of some thin material, either white or plain blue, black or brown in colour, somewhere within easy reach of the Bodhi-Mandala, which they don over their ordinary clothes before entering the shrine for a session, and remove on emerging afterwards. Their doing this should not be mistaken for a frivolous fondness for dressing up to add consequence to their appearance, as wearing a special robe during cultivation serves a yogic purpose. Psychologically it symbolises the apartness of what takes place in the Bodhi-Mandala from the sometimes turgid and negative emotions inextricably bound up with everyday affairs conducted beyond the Bodhi-Mandala's peaceful bounds; thus it helps to maintain what is known as ritual purity. Furthermore, as a notable addition to the gracefulness and dignity of prostrations and other yogic movements, it contributes to the beauty and grace that should characterise every aspect of yogic cultivation, making it 'pleasing to gods and men', that is to say lovely and immaculate.

In China and Tibet Buddhists were fond of making pilgrimages involving journeys on foot that might take several days, or even several months or years. Occasionally, a pilgrim would undertake to make such a journey stopping after every three steps to prostrate himself to the ground. Hsü Yün, the most noted Ch'an Master of the present century, once travelled in this manner all the way from a point on the South China coast just opposite P'u-t'o Island (sacred to the Bodhisattva Kuan Yin) to Mount Wu T'ai in northern China (sacred to the Bodhisattva Manjusri, Embodiment of Wisdom) – a distance of a thousand miles as the crow flies and much longer by the shortest practicable route. So athletic was this master and so accustomed to making prostrations that, bowing to the earth after every three steps, he accomplished the journey within two years. Recently, two American disciples of Master Hsüan Hua progressed in the same manner from Los Angeles to the City of Ten Thousand Buddhas established a few years ago in Ukaiya, a hundred miles or so to the north of San Francisco, their object being to make fruitful aspirations for world peace. Though I, personally, would hesitate to recommend such an extreme form of piety on that scale, I have observed that some Western adepts do find the performance of challenging feats inspiring, so the following modified form of the three-steps-one-prostration practice may be found acceptable. There are already some Western Buddhist communities where the custom of perambulating, say, the top of a small mountain is observed on certain days of the year, with those taking part continuously reciting a mantra or a chanted invocation as they walk. It might be appropriate on such an occasion for a procession of dedicated adepts to spend an afternoon, or the best part of a whole day, perambulating the chosen place, while chanting invocations to Kuan Yin and prostrating themselves at every three steps. The words 'Namo Mahā karunā Avalokiteśvara Bodhisattva' (Homage to the Infinitely Compassionate Kuan Yin Bodhisattva) could be set to a tune that would govern the rhythm of taking three paces forward, making a full prostration, rising, taking three more paces forward, and so on. The chanters would concentrate throughout the practice on the generation of bodhi-citta, that is of an immaculate mind filled with the wisdom beyond thought and with infinite compassion. Kuan Yin, the embodiment of the wisdom-compassion energy latent within Mind, would, in response to so powerful an invocation, certainly arise in the minds of those taking part and confer augmented wisdom and compassion that would have lasting results for all who perform the practice with undeviating concentration and sincerity.

(d) SITTING

There is no need to repeat here the instructions for sitting given in section I, B, 2, (b), to which readers should now refer. All that is said there about posture, meditation cushions, garments, etc., applies equally to Buddhist meditation, except that Buddhist masters tend to be stricter than most Taoists as to posture, preferring the full lotus or half-lotus posture to any others, if the meditators are capable of maintaining one of these. Moreover, the position of the hands is different. Usually the left hand lies palm-upward on the lap, with the right hand, also held palm-upward, resting upon it in such a way that the tips of the thumbs touch each other to facilitate the circulation of *ch'i*.

During long sessions, if some refeshment or a remedy for drowsiness was needed, it was customary in China to drink rather strong (milkless and sugarless) green tea. Of the kinds available in the China-towns of the West, the most suitable for this purpose is known as 'Iron Kuan Yin', this being the name of the place in South China where it is grown. (Properly called *T'ieh Kuan Yin ch'a*, it is known to the Cantonese shopkeepers there as *Tit Gwoon-Yam*, of which the last syllable rhymes with the English word 'gum'.) Traditionally it was served in handleless cups, both teapot and cups having generally been chosen for their austere simplicity of form and lack of distracting decoration. Brewed in advance, the tea was kept hot by placing the pot in a lidded basket with a thickly quilted cloth lining. It is said that the elaborate tea ceremony evolved in Japan had its origin in the drinking of tea by Ch'an monks in Chinese monasteries during the intervals punctuating their long meditation ceremonies. Their manner of serving and drinking it did follow a prescribed ritual, but one utterly simple in comparison with the Japanese *cha no yu* in its present form and, as the tea was served in the meditation hall, silence naturally prevailed.

(e) BREATHING

There is a wide range of Buddhist meditational techniques concerned with breathing, their purpose being both to calm the restless waves of thought so as to induce one-pointedness of mind, and to facilitate the inflow of *ch'i* which, in Sanskrit, is called *prana*. The more advanced techniques involve some danger to health and should be studied under the supervision of an accomplished teacher, but even the simple ones that require no supervision can be very effective. These are normally performed while sitting in meditation posture.

Buddhists, no less than Taoists, favour the technique described in I, B, 2, (c) above, which consists of taking evenly spaced inhalations and exhalations during which awareness is concentrated upon the silent passage of the breath as it passes in and out of the nostrils. This can be performed as an exercise on its own, but is chiefly used during a space of five or ten minutes for stilling the mind in preparation for some other contemplative practice; moreover, many meditators like to revert to it for a few minutes at the end of their main practice.

A variation of this method, which may also be used either on its own or else as a preliminary to some other practice, is to fix the awareness upon a silent counting of each inhalation-cum-exhalation, the count being from one to ten and repeated for as long as seems desirable. This is particularly suitable for beginners who find difficulty in keeping their awareness fixed for more than a few moments, because the need to keep a count prevents the mind from wandering. A further variant is to substitute for the counting mental repetition of the words 'i...n' and 'ou...t', which are prolonged to fit the length of each inhalation or exhalation. The words should not be spoken, but occur in the mind as a rhythmic accompaniment to the breathing upon which the awareness is centred. This latter variant can also be performed at any time throughout the day, whether one happens to be walking, standing, sitting or lying; whenever the adept is conscious of the arising of anger or of some other unwholesome state of mind, he should withdraw his attention from the circumstances that have caused it to arise, carefully regulate his breathing and attend solely to his silent repetition of the words 'in' and 'out'. Psychologically this will distract him from the unwholesome emotion; physiologically, by leading to slow, harmonious and relatively deep breathing, it will facilitate an influx of *ch'i* that will counteract the physiological processes to which the emotion gives rise, thus causing it to subside. Yet another use of this variant is to still the mind when excitement or unwholesome emotions of any kind make it difficult to fall asleep at the customary time.

The interrelated techniques discussed in the previous two paragraphs may all be further varied in the following way. Instead of maintaining the same rhythm of inhalation and exhalation without change for the duration of the exercise, one may begin by taking relatively short breaths and then gradually lengthen them until they become unusually deep and long-sustained, but inhalation and exhalation should still be evenly balanced and the breathing remain absolutely silent. (See also II, B, 4, (b) below for a different method of combining breathing with awareness.)

One may feel, perhaps, that the exercises just described, though well suited to beginners, are disappointingly elementary, and look forward to discarding them in favour of more advanced techniques. This, I think, would be a wrong attitude. Not only do advanced breathing practices involve some danger and require qualified supervision that must be preceded, in the case of Tibetan techniques, by an initiation sometimes difficult to obtain; but also those already set forth are by no means suited only to beginners; on the contrary, they are used by many yogins at all stages of the Way. A supposition to the contrary arises from failure to understand the deeper implications of simple breath watching and breath control. These are as follows: (i) Many of the body's functions are affected by the nature of one's breathing; when breathing, after the conscious control given to it by the adept initially, becomes naturally rhythmic, harmonious and not too shallow, the whole functioning of the body is brought to a state of calm equilibrium, and this assists the mind to achieve a more nearly permanent stillness accompanied by habitual serenity. (ii) Breathing, being an activity that proceeds involuntarily but yet can at any moment be brought under conscious control, pertains to the threshold between the conscious and subconscious levels of being. The meditator in seeking to expand his consciousness depends, therefore, on controlled breathing to open the gates to those deeper levels not ordinarily within its scope. (iii) Breath is the vehicle by means of which *ch'i* or cosmic vitality penetrates the human body. When breathing is harmonious and has become habitually deeper than that of an uninstructed man, the influx and circulation of *ch'i* throughout the body is augmented and becomes more regularly sustained, being less subject to unconscious blockage. Though this is not the place to go into the concept of a 'breath-body' as a counterpart of the physical body, that being a matter with which only advanced yogins need be concerned, it is pertinent to observe here that practice in simple awareness and control of the breathing process constitutes admirable training in preparation for the time when a teacher of advanced yoga is encountered. If, by that time, the adept has so mastered the technique of correct breathing that it has become for him normal and spontaneous, he will be able to respond to further teaching much more promptly and effectively.

When planning this book, I originally intended to include some account of the Nine Breaths technique well known to yogins; but, on reflection, I realised that this is rarely taught – if ever – without prior initiation, so I deleted it from the proposed contents. I mention it here as something that the adept may hope to learn sooner or later from a qualified Tibetan lama upon request. In the meanwhile, he will do well to learn to breathe at all times more deeply and in a more regulated manner than hitherto. The effects will be far-reaching and, as I have said, he will be laying a foundation for advanced breathing yoga, as well as bringing about a marked improvement to his general health.

(f) STILLNESS

It is because the mind, deluded by false concepts arising from the imperfect or limited functioning of sense perception, has come to resemble an ocean forever at the mercy of shifting winds and currents that contemplative meditation is so essential to the winning of Enlightenment. Until the waves of idle thought subside, there is scant possibility of achieving intuitive perception of the true face of reality. Buddhists, Taoists, mystics of all faiths are alike in proclaiming the wisdom of striving for mental stillness – though striving is perhaps a misleading word, as stillness depends on cessation rather than activity. Perfect mental stillness, sustained over a period of some minutes or much longer, is not infrequently termed objectless awareness; but, as the Lama Govinda has wisely pointed out in a recent book, true objectless awareness is impossible, since awareness by its very nature has to be awareness of something.

One makes a start by seeking one-pointedness of mind; that is to say the waves of thought are caused gently to subside by focusing the mind unwaveringly upon a single object. Initially, this may be anything at all – an actual object such as a steady point of light; an imagined object, such as a *bija-mantra* (consisting of one glowing syllable), or else, say, a cross or swastika visualised as being in front of one on a level with the eyes; a sensation such as the inhalation and exhalation of breath, or the pulsing of the blood; a part of the body, such as the Mysterious Gate lying behind the mid-point between the eyes, or the Fire Centre on a level with the navel; and so on, for there is no end to the list. At a later stage, awareness becomes very nearly objectless like the beam of a bright lantern shining upon a limitless expanse of immaculate snow; and, still later, intuition of the immeasurable stillness lying at the heart of cosmic movement blossoms. Beyond this lie realms beyond all power of description and, returning thence, the meditator will have no way to describe the content of his awareness during the mind-shattering experience of his sojourn there. Meanwhile, at quite an early stage, visions may occur of brilliant lights, heavenly beings and so forth, but these should not be allowed to distract the attention; for, like ordinary objects in the meditator's immediate environment, they are potential disturbers of his inner stillness – not to be rudely shunned or cast out, but quietly dismissed from the focus of his attention like any other wandering thoughts that may arise.

Unwavering contemplation of any single object or phenomenon is a good way of attaining inner stillness – not total blankness (which is undesirable) but sustained one-pointedness. This practice may at first seem unrewarding and give rise to boredom, but with the dawning of stillness will come sensations of joyous tranquillity sometimes amounting to bliss. Yet even these may constitute distractions, so one should not dwell on them, but just persist in maintaining stillness for its own sake.

Stillness, stillness, stillness! Herein lies the key to true success in yogic contemplation. Stillness opens up the mind to mystery upon mystery, culminating in Enlightenment itself.

(g) A STORY

A certain youth, on hearing of the Way, decided to pursue it at all costs. Leaving home, he shaved his head and went to study under a solitary old monk who inhabited a small and little-known temple in the neighbourhood of Fêng T'ai, near Peking. In due course, the young man went off to the famous Chieh T'ai Monastery in the Western Hills to receive ordination and master between two and three hundred monastic precepts, which he henceforth observed most scrupulously. Thereafter he became a wandering monk, searching everywhere for new sources of wisdom. Travelling through the lonely fastnesses in the neighbourhood of the Great Wall, he ascended Mount Wu T'ai, where some three hundred temples were clustered on a flowery plateau or clung to the slopes and summits of its five tall peaks. Staying there for above two years, he received instruction from Chinese, Mongolian and even Tibetan teachers in the mysteries of esoteric Buddhism. Next he trudged over hundreds of miles to sacred Mount Chiu Hua in the province of Anhui, often sleeping under the frosty stars with scant protection from the autumn winds and having little to eat but a bowlful of millet gruel or a couple of coarse maize rolls. There he studied in one of the smaller temples where there dwelt at that time a sage highly skilled in Ch'an (Zen) meditation, from whom he acquired much more than the rudiments of Ch'an technique. Thence, he walked southwards for many weeks until he came to the Yangtse River and embarked as a deck passenger on a large wooden junk that had to be hauled against a strong current by teams of men who, straining at the ropes, pressed forward with their bodies bent low along the rocky shore. Oppressed by the sticky climate in that region, he passed day after day in study and meditation until at last they reached Chia Ting, whence another and smaller junk took him up a tributary river to the foot of mighty Mount Omei. Undeterred by stories of the revenge taken by the monkeys on its forested slopes against travellers who treated them discourteously, he toiled up what must surely be the tallest staircase in the world, meeting a few monkeys but saluting them kindly with appropriate words from the Buddhist sutras. On the lofty summit of this mountain, he passed some months studying the Hua Yen doctrine from a scholarly monk who expounded the teaching that every object, be it as small as the tip of a fine hair, contains within itself the entire cosmos. Thus the young monk became acquainted with a profound and subtle philosophy.

Feeling sadly as far from Enlightenment as ever, he boarded another vessel and was carried swiftly down river to the port of

Shanghai, whence he proceeded on foot to a point on the South China coast opposite the sea-girt island of Pʻu-tʻo, sacred to the Bodhisattva Kuan Yin. There he crossed what was believed to be a dragon-haunted ocean during weather that caused all the passengers to suffer cruelly from seasickness, and came at last to the island where he was to spend the next five years immersed in the practices of the Pure Land school of Buddhism. Twice he was rewarded with fleeting visions of the Bodhisattva in the Chʻao-yang cave, but not with anything resembling Enlightenment. Not knowing where else to go in search of wisdom, he returned to the mainland and trudged northward for many months until he arrived exhausted at the little temple near Fêng Tʻai whence his long and arduous journey had begun some ten years earlier.

That same old solitary monk, the very first of his innumerable teachers, still dwelt there, so he received the warm welcome for which he had been longing, his host being only too happy to listen for days on end to a full recital of his wanderings.

'Wonderful!' exclaimed the old man, after hearing about all the famous monks under whom his pupil had studied and the details of the teachings they had imparted. 'Though you were once my own little disciple, I now intend to prostrate myself before you, knowing that by now you must certainly have become a Bodhisattva!' So saying, he rose swiftly to his feet.

'No, no!' implored the younger man, leaping up just in time to prevent his former teacher from falling to his knees. 'It would be a shame to permit Your Reverence to suppose anything of that kind. True, I have acquired a great deal of knowledge and read thousands of volumes since last we met, besides listening attentively to sermons without number, but I am such a stupid fellow that what I have learnt amounts to nothing in terms of wisdom. Of that precious commodity I do not have enough to make a thin coating for the smallest of copper coins.'

'So that's how it is!' exclaimed the elder, a smile hovering on his lips. 'Well, to tell you the truth, I am not altogether surprised. I wonder if you happened to dip into the small volume I gave you as a parting present before you went off to the Western Hills to receive ordination?'

'Alas, no', replied the other shamefacedly. 'You see, in those days my education was still limited and I could not make head or tail of the ancient characters in which that copy of the *Tao Tê Ching* was printed.'

'Never mind', smiled the old monk. 'As it happens, I have here a tattered copy of the same work printed in ordinary characters, and you are now learned enough to expound the full meaning to me – that is certain. Here, turn to section 47 and read the words aloud.'

Obediently the wandering monk read out: 'Without leaving the house, one may know all there is in heaven and earth. Without peeping from the window, one may see the ways of heaven. Those who go out learn less and less the more they travel. Wherefore does the Sage know all without going anywhere, see all without looking, do nothing and achieve [the Goal]!'

'Do you understand?' cried the old man, fixing his eyes on his erstwhile pupil. 'Ah, what a waste of effort! What hardships suffered for nothing! How the orations of a hundred wordy masters must have tired your ears! The Goal can be attained right here. Just close the doors of the senses and cultivate stillness. There is really no more to be said.'

Now a sudden illumination burst upon his pupil, who fell to his knees and began beating his head on the stone flags at the old man's feet, crying: 'Good, good. I have at last found my true master!'

'Where, where?' cried the old man warily and sprang lightly to his feet. 'Does he stand here before you? Or do you mean he is here in this book?'

'No!' replied the young monk joyfully. 'He is much closer than that. He has been right here inside me since the very beginning, but hidden by the stinking mists and opaque miasmas of my own stupid thoughts and ambitions.'

'Just so,' laughed the other, slapping himself with joy. 'What a pity you did not ask me where to find him, before hurrying off on that long journey!'

3

Practices Involving Body, Speech and Mind

(a) THE THREE REFUGES

This is a basic rite common in all Buddhist countries. Indeed, it is a means of formally becoming a Buddhist, which can be done simply by pronouncing the formula of taking refuge in the Triple˚Gem thrice with sincerity, whether in public or alone. Thus, anyone drawn by the teaching of the Enlightened One can become a Buddhist without further ado. Furthermore, this formula and the brief ritual that commonly accompanies it are employed by serious Buddhists at least once every day of their lives, and commonly used as a prologue to every meditation session. It is the modern fashion in the West to be averse to rites and ceremonies; though why this should be is hard to say, as they have been deemed beautiful and meaningful by man through all the centuries since the dawn of history – in Asia, Africa, Amerind America, and in Europe whether in Greek and Roman times, or during the medieval and Renaissance periods and much later; besides, they would provide a pleasant antidote to the drabness of modern life – as evidenced by such phenomena as the delight afforded to the crowds at Disneyland by the splendid nightly processions. Like singing and dancing, rites are a means for man to express his heartfelt aspirations. Yogically, the importance of the one now to be described is that it is a remedy to egotistic self-satisfaction and the consequent harmful enlargement of ego-delusion that may otherwise result from success in meditation. It should not be difficult for people who accept the military necessity of saluting officers and are prepared to bow to the illustrious dead during ceremonies performed at a cenotaph to show even greater respect to that fount of wisdom, compassion and peace known to Buddhists as the 'Teacher of Gods and Men' and to the whole world as the Enlightened One.

In its simplest form, the rite consists of repeating slowly and

thoughtfully, three times in succession, the formula: 'I go for refuge
to the Buddha. I go for refuge to the Dharma. I go for refuge to the
Sangha.' The full implication of these words is something like:
'Having faith in the Enlightened One, his Teaching and the Community of beings who practise it, I intend henceforth to live by that
teaching and work towards ultimately attaining liberation through
Buddha-like Enlightenment.' A triple repetition of the formula is
sufficient in itself, but it has been customary to start by lighting a stick
of incense and to prostrate oneself before an image or statue of the
Buddha once after reciting each of the constituent sentences. Thus,
nine prostrations are made in all during the threefold utterance of the
whole formula. Each of the sentences is intoned while standing or
kneeling, and the prostration follows immediately.

At least once a day, Chinese Buddhists recite the formula in an
amplified form, a chant which includes expressions of aspiration for
the welfare of all sentient beings, of which the following is a translation:

> *I go for refuge to the Buddha,*
> *Desiring that all sentient beings,*
> *By cleaving to the lofty Way,*
> *May attain to wisdom unexcelled.*

> *I go for refuge to the Dharma,*
> *Desiring that all sentient beings,*
> *By deep study of the sacred writings,*
> *May attain to knowledge ocean-wide.*

> *I go for refuge to the Sangha,*
> *Desiring that all sentient beings,*
> *United by a single cause,*
> *Free from all impediment,*
> *May reverence the sacred Order.*

The Chinese original is worded more beautifully, but it is never easy
to put Chinese into something like metrical English without departing
somewhat from the original. The Chinese tune to which the words are
sung is probably of distant Indian origin and hauntingly beautiful, but
exceptionally difficult to render in Western notation; besides, it
would not fit the English words. Any simple, yet solemn tune
somewhere between singing and chanting will do. The Chinese
custom is to stand with the hands placed palm to palm before the
breast for the first two lines of each verse and then prostrate oneself

swiftly so that the head reaches the floor (or meditation cushion) just before the verse ends. A pause before the next verse begins makes it possible to regain the standing position in good time. During the very long meditation sessions that are held in Chinese temples from time to time (with up to eighteen hours of meditation every day), rituals of this kind help to mitigate the effects of prolonged sitting.

(b) BOWING WITH CHANT

This practice is rather similar to the one just described, in that it inculcates feelings of reverence and awe for the greater-than-self and counteracts egotistic self-esteem. In this case, however, a brief formula is intoned many hundreds or thousands of times in succession, thus adding to its psychological effect as an approach to inner stillness. When a single adept performs this rite, he sinks to his knees and touches his head to the ground during each alternate invocation, which is sufficiently prolonged to permit that, and rises slowly to an erect position, hands palm to palm before his chest, during the intervening repetitions. If a number of people perform it jointly, they divide into two groups, one to the left of the Buddha image with their toes pointing towards meditation cushions spread out in rows at suitable distances from each other to allow free, uncrowded movement, the other group to the right. If any particular person is officiating, he may stand alone in the space between the two groups. During the initial chanting of the invocation, one group remains standing, while the other performs a prostration. Thereafter, as one group goes down the other rises and this alternation continues until the end, when one group remains standing while the other rises. When the two groups are able to prostrate themselves gracefully, the sight is impressive, especially if all are wearing ankle-length robes.

The words of the chant are very simple. They should be intoned slowly with the individual syllables prolonged so as to allow time for those bowing down and those rising to their feet to accomplish their movements smoothly. The words most often used are: *Namu Pên-shih Shih-chia-mo-ni Fu* in Chinese, or 'Homage to the Founding Teacher Shakyamuni Buddha' in English. Perhaps the Sanskrit equivalent, *Namu Upādhyāya Śākyamuni Buddha*, would sound more euphonious and be easier to chant melodiously. ('Ś' has the sound of 'Sh'.) All the syllables are chanted on the same note, except for the last three. Of these the 'ni' starts on the same note and then rises a semi-tone above it, and the syllables 'Buddha' are chanted a full tone below the rest.

The whole can thus be symbolised thus:

Na–a–a–mu–u Oo–padh–ya–ya Shakya–mu–u– ni–i Buddha–a

When healing practice based on contemplation of the Bodhisattva Kuan Yin is being performed (see II, B, 5, (a)–(c)), the words are *Namu Ta-pei Kuan-shih-yin P'u-sa* or 'Homage to the Compassionate Kuan Shih Yin Bodhisattva' or *Namu Mahā-karunā Avalokiteśvara Bodhisattva.* The tune could be symbolised:

Na–a–a–mu–u   Ma–ha–a–ka–ru–u–na–a   Avalokiteśva–a–ra

Bodhi–sa–at–va–a

If the Chinese chant, indicated with lines long and short to suggest syllable length, accents to show stress and higher or lower lines towards the end to indicate half a tone higher or a full tone lower than the rest (in a minor key), is difficult to comprehend, or if it does not sound inspiring or conduce to inner stillness, any rather similar chant in a minor key and any altered spacing will do well.

(c) MANTRAS, MUDRĀS AND MENTALLY CREATED OFFERINGS

Mantras are powerful utterances that do not necessarily yield any obvious verbal meaning. Not to be confused with magic spells, they are strings of sound that owe their power to psychic affinities – a subject too complicated to be gone into in a few words, but dealt with to the best of my ability in a work called *Mantras: Words of Power* (published by Allen & Unwin in the United Kingdom and by Shambhala Press in the United States). Perhaps there can never be a full explanation of how they operate; that they are immensely effective is warrant enough for uttering them. Generally mantras are not disclosed to non-initiates, as they have to be studied under a qualified teacher, but the mantra known as the 'Mani' that is explained below is now so widely known that yogic secrecy applies to it no longer. Though it is best to seek initiation into its multifold uses, it can be effectively employed without a teacher, provided that it is properly *mastered*, that is to say repeated many hundreds or thousands of times a day over a considerable period with absolute sincerity by an adept who is constantly striving to behave towards other beings with deep compassion. The offering mantras, also explained below, do not absolutely require initiation for their effective use.

Mudrās are sacred gestures made with the hands, which similarly owe their power to affinity with psychic forces. The same restrictions apply to them as to mantras, with only a few exceptions.

Mentally created offerings are offerings in the form of one, seven or eight bowls of pure, fresh water (or even offerings present only as ideas in the adept's mind) that can be converted into all sorts of beautiful and precious substances on a vast cosmic scale by the power of mind. When a yogic rite involving them is to be performed, if actual offerings are available, that is best; otherwise, a bowl or bowls of water or mental images of what are required can be substituted. Real offerings, those symbolised by pure water and those which exist only as mental images can all be beautiful and multiplied by the power of mind, which is paramount in all forms of yogic cultivation. Like other ritualistic forms, offerings are primarily beneficial in that they are productive of certain states of mind; it is not to be supposed that the Buddhas and Bodhisattvas demand or stand in need of them, still less that they exact them from their devotees on pain of dire displeasure! Such concepts are alien to Buddhism.

It is by the use of mudrās, mantras and mental visualisations that the three faculties of body, speech and mind can be employed simultaneously for yogic purposes.

The mantra known as the 'Mani' consists of six Sanskrit syllables, namely *OṀ MĀNI PADMÉ HŪṀ*, of which *PADMÉ* is very commonly pronounced 'BEMÉ'; *MĀ* rhymes with the first syllable of 'father'; *NI* is pronounced like the English word 'knee'; *PAD* more or less rhymes with 'bud' as pronounced in southern England; *MÉ* rhymes with 'may'; *HŪṀ* rhymes with 'room' pronounced rather shortly. The syllable *HŪṀ* itself is often sustained for a long time while intoning the mantra; what I mean is that the vowel itself is shorter than in the English word 'loom' for example. If the varient *BEMÉ* is used, it rhymes with 'bay-may'. This is the mantra associated with the Bodhisattva of Compassion, Avalokiteśvara (Chinese, Kuan Yin; Tibetan, Chenresigs). Besides being suitable for use in the healing practices set forth in section II, B, 6, (b)–(d), it has a powerful effect in achieving stillness, peace of mind, fearlessness in the face of danger, etc.; moreover, it can banish or completely transform baneful visions or evil dreams, once one has learnt how to resort to it during moments of stress or while asleep; above all, it is a means of evoking compassion for oneself and especially for other beings. However, it becomes fully effective only after it has been mastered by frequent repetition during which the compassionate Bodhisattva is invoked with heartfelt fervour and clearly visualised. Those bent on mastering the Mani for use in times of stress and on behalf of suffering beings should repeat it thousands of times a day over a long period and, thereafter, do so as frequently as possible for as long as they live, though never when their minds are entertaining thoughts at odds with or extraneous to the vital principle of compassion embodied in Kuan Yin. Properly mastered, it is one of the most fruitful of all yogic devices for dealing with anxiety, fear, panic and hysteria, and for helping beings in urgent need, as well as for transmuting negative passions such as envy, jealousy, or anger into joyous tranquillity.

In many Asian countries, a string of 108 beads (sometimes with strings of tiny metal discs attached for recording counts of a hundred or a thousand) is used as a tally by adepts who have set themselves to repeat the Mani so many hundred, thousand or tens of thousands of times with a given period. If a string of beads of this kind is hard to come by, one can instead decide to spend so many minutes or hours a day on reciting the Mani in order to master it, in which case no tally is required. However, it is fruitless to do this, unless one is forever trying one's utmost to be compassionate in thought, word and deed towards all kinds of beings, not excluding poisonous reptiles and insects. To cause harm wittingly to any sentient being should be unthinkable. Thus sports like hunting, shooting and fishing must be totally eschewed, otherwise yogic practice becomes an impious farce.

The mantras and mudrās for the offerings that are required during a great many yogic rites are as follows. During their use, the mind should be employed in visualising images of each offering in a form as magnificent and beautiful as possible.

Water for the face *OṀ ARGHAM AH HŪṀ* Hands held out at breast level in such a manner as to form the likeness of a shallow bowl, of which part of the rim consists of the thumbs resting upon the gently curving fingers.

Water for bathing *OṀ PADYAM AH HŪṀ* Hands held out separately at breast level, each with the first two fingers

		extended, the other two folded and held down by the thumb. The projecting fingers of each hand are caused to revolve round those of the other hand thrice, to suggest moving water.
Flowers	OṀ PUSHPÉ AH HŪṀ	Hands held palm to palm at breast level in an attitude of prayer, but with the fingers interlaced to form a single line of upward pointing finger tips. The hands, though joined at the finger-tips and just above the wrists, arch away from each other in the middle to suggest the shape of a lotus bud. The thumbs, rising vertically side by side, enclose the near end of the bud.
Incense	OṀ DHUPÉ AH HŪṀ	Hands held back to back at breast level with the sky-ward pointing fingers inter-laced (thumbs held close to the forefingers) to suggest incense sticks rising from a censer.
Lamps	OṀ ALOKÉ AH HŪṀ	Hands held out palms upward and separate from each other at breast level, fingers tightly curled so that the nails point down with their surfaces facing the breast, upward-pointing thumbs erect with their bases pushed towards the centre of the palm, to suggest wicks rising from the centre of a saucer of oil.
Perfumed water	OṀ GANDHÉ AH HŪṀ	Left hand held horizontally at breast level, palm upward, fingertips point-ing away from the body,

| | | thumb curved to rest on the palm. Right hand held vertically, thumb curved as above, with the base of the palm lightly resting on the extreme edge of the left hand, to represent a ewer standing by a flat saucerlike receptacle. |
| Pure food (e.g., excellent fruits) | *OṀ NAIVIDHÉ AH HŪṀ* | Hands forming a bowl exactly as for the first mudrā, except that the thumbs curl inwards and rest on the palms, to suggest a shallow bowl containing pure food. |

Each of these mudrās, during the performance of which the mantras are said, is preceded by a gesture made by crossing the right wrist over the left in front of the breast, so that the fingers of the right hand point towards the left shoulder, those of the left hand towards the right shoulder, and simultaneously producing a clicking sound by pressing the tips of the middle fingers hard against the thumb tips and bringing them down forcefully to smack against the palms.

Immediately after each mudrā, the same clicking gesture is made, but with the left wrist outside the right.

Meanwhile, one visualises a spirit attendant appearing in response to the first click, who stands ready to receive the offering symbolised by the immediately following mudrā. The second click dispatches this attendant to lay the offering in front of the Buddha or Bodhisattva, now visualised as a living being. The sequence is conveyed by the following diagram, in which circles labelled R and L stand respectively for clicks made with the right or left wrist outward, and squares (each containing the initial letter of the appropriate offering) stand for the mudrās:

R⬜L R⬜L R⬜L R⬜L R⬜L R⬜L R⬜L
○W○ ○W○ ○F○ ○I○ ○L○ ○P○ ○F○

The underlying principle is that, whether one uses actual bowls of offerings, or seven bowls of water to represent them, or just visualises the offerings as lying before one, one can, by reciting the mantras and forming the appropriate mudrās accompanied by intense visualisation, give vast, cosmic dimensions to the offerings, endow them with mind-boggling beauty and serve them in exquisitely adorned bowls of solid gold inlaid with precious gems. This sequence of offerings originated in India and may have been used in ancient times for the worship of anthropomorphic Hindu deities, which would account for the nature of the substances offered. As we have seen, it was the Buddhist custom to adapt the pre-Buddhist iconography and rites prevalent in various countries for use in a Buddhist context. For the last two thousand years or so, the seven offerings (or sometimes eight, with music symbolised by conch-shells added) have been used mainly as a prelude to various tantric rituals that cannot under any circumstances be performed prior to initiation. The inclusion of these mundras in this book is for several reasons. First, they are among the very few that can be taught without prior initiation. Second, they illustrate how, in tantric practice, acts of body, speech and mind are combined. Third, this rite can be of practical use as a prelude to the cleansing and healing yogas described in a later section. In this regard, it must again be emphasised that the Celestial Buddhas and Bodhisattvas are not thought to stand in need of offerings; yet it is yogically desirable that the adept use this means of generating a spirit of reverence and awe. To some people, the ritual may seem meaningless, in which case it is better to omit it; for others, it will be highly effective in stimulating a yogic state of mind, especially in preparation for cleansing and healing yogas.

Ritual gestures are, after all, used by almost everybody to generate or symbolise appropriate states of mind, as when one salutes the flag, ceremoniously removes one's hat, kneels in church, shakes hands, performs masonic rites, wears academic robes to bestow or receive a university degree, and so on. Their universality indicates that they fulfil a human need. (Those extreme Protestants who made a point of not kneeling in church do in fact make a ritual of *not kneeling*!) At some seminars in North America, T'ai Chi Master Huang Chung-liang (Al Huang) wove the offering mudrās into a very beautiful sacred dance. Dancing is, of course, another very ancient way of expressing profound reverence to that which is greater than self, for example to the Tao as the life-force animating all beings, or to the Bodhisattvas or psychic embodiments of the principles of wisdom and compassion.

The main point to remember is that mantras and mudrās should be accompanied by intense visualisation. One should learn to 'see' the jewelled bowls of offerings and their lovely contents, the coming and going of spirit attendants dressed in shining silken robes, and the acceptance of the offerings by a being whose mien betokens glorious serenity and sweet compassion, as clearly as if all these happenings were right before the eyes.

(d) A STORY

A certain yogin dwelt in a cave close to the shores of the Blue Lake (Kokonor) in the beautiful flower-carpeted wilderness which forms a frontier region on the borders of China, Mongolia and Tibet. There he had lived in solitude for seven years, being rarely seen and even more rarely holding converse with the villagers who faithfully came each day with offerings of food and other necessities to supply his meagre wants. His reputation for unblemished sanctity had spread far and wide. One day, a Chinese official on a tour of inspection in that region halted his cavalcade not far from the yogin's cave and, dismounting, climbed alone to its mouth. Seeing nothing but a few ragged sheep-skins, an old bronze kettle, the implements for making a charcoal fire to brew tea, and a few primitive eating utensils, where he had expected to come upon the yogin himself, he raised his voice and cried: 'Holy One, Holy One, this insignificant person craves audience.'

'Who is it?' These words, pronounced in a ringing voice, came from the shadowed depths beyond.

'My humble surname is Han. I am touring the district as representative of the Governor of Ch'ing Hai, and have stopped over to pay my respects to you.'

'What can an exalted personage such as Your Honour want with an ignorant old fellow like me?' replied the voice.

'Ah, no ceremony, I beg. Your Reverence's reputation resounds throughout the district. How can I not have much to learn from you? Please disregard my unworthy rank and receive me as a simple person much in need of wisdom.'

Something moved in the darkness and the inspector-general now beheld a thin old man clad in a shabby bronze-coloured robe, whose sparse, unkempt hair hung loosely to his shoulders. Inviting his guest to sit down upon a pile of sheepskin bedding, the old man busied himself with the charcoal stove and soon a tea-kettle was on the boil.

'Holy One,' inquired the official at length, 'do you not feel lonely here, so far from the sound of human voices?'

'*Lonely*!' exclaimed the hermit, obviously astounded. 'No, no, no. I am seldom alone. From dawn to midnight, my cave is thronged with visitors.'

'I see no sign of them,' answered Han, wondering whether the old fellow had all his wits about him.

'Naturally, Sir. Naturally. The throngs of beings are mental creations, invisible to others.'

'Mental creations? How, then, can they banish loneliness? I understand that you *see* them, but since they cannot converse . . .'

'Indeed they converse with me night and day, and have taught me innumerable wonderful and sacred things. How not?'

'Surely creations of your mind can do no more than tell you what you already know?'

At this the old hermit appeared so overcome with astonishment as to be at a loss for words. After a long pause, he said: 'It is from incomparable Mind, vaster than a billion billion chiliocosms, that these beings are generated. Wherefore a space of innumerable aeons would be too short to exhaust their teaching. The wisdom of all the sages known to this world does not encompass more than a hair's tip of the whole.'

An orthodox Confucian by upbringing, the learned inspector-general felt himself reel back from these immensities as from a limitless abyss. Aware that such a dialogue could proceed no further without his becoming lost amidst uncharted seas, he sought to end it by exclaiming: 'Admirable! Admirable! Most deeply do I regret that my studies have not equipped me to hear the converse of your spiritual masters!'

Struck by his guest's sincerity and not a little surprised to find humility in a personage whose rank proclaimed him to be a scholar of high distinction, the hermit replied: 'Permit me to try to communicate my experience to Your Excellency.'

To this Han joyfully agreed and the old man, taking up the lotus posture, began intoning some mantras, his hands meanwhile weaving a series of intricate gestures that merged one into another too swiftly for the Confucian to distinguish them individually. Presently the gestures ceased, but the mantric hum proceeding from the other's lips increased in volume until the cave resounded as though it were situated atop a high mountain pass, wide open to a great wind that came rushing in and battering against the walls. Simultaneously, the darkness was dispelled by a soft light that, growing ever more brilliant and illumining every nook and cranny, revealed a host of lovely beings clad in shimmering garments of silken gauze. From within these beings now shone forth a radiance that produced a multicoloured flame-like aura which enveloped the entire assembly of seated figures rising tier upon tier to a height many times greater than that of the cave itself, for the rocky ceiling was no longer to be seen.

'Who can they be?' wondered the amazed Confucian, who could put no questions to his new friend for as long as the torrent of mantric sound proceeding from his lips continued. Instantly, however, the answer flashed into his mind as though spoken by the hermit: 'These are the Teachers of my line, extending backwards through the ages to the Enlightened One himself, whom you see seated above the Eight Celestial Bodhisattvas and other exalted beings.'

Looking up to the apex of that shining pyramid of beings, Han made out the topmost figure to be Shakyamuni Buddha, Teacher of Gods and Men, whose gentle smile and half-closed eyes proclaimed the rapturous bliss of *samadhi*.

'Were one of these majestic beings to speak at length,' reflected the Confucian scholar, 'I should know whether the substance of his words sprang from the content of my own mind or from some other source, and thus discover the answer to my question about gaining knowledge from mentally created beings.'

No sooner had this entered his mind than a voice proclaimed in mellifluous accents: 'Our speech has no relation to mere learning, yet you may truly call it a reflection of your own mind, there being no distinction between the minds of sentient beings and boundless Mind, other than the illusory barrier arising from ignorance of the unity of one and all. How can your mind and Mind be two, since both share the true nature of the void?'

Much else followed before the discourse ceased, the radiance faded and the stream of mantric sound subsided into stillness, leaving the old hermit rapt, as the Buddha had been, in the bliss of *samadhi*. Han's question had been answered; for, like most Confucian scholars, he had not been familiar with the doctrine of the One Mind, which was therefore new to him and could not have been propounded by what he had always taken to be his own mind – viewed as a personal possession having nothing in common with other minds or with what he had now learnt to call Mind as a synonym for the Tao, the Void, Reality.

As the hermit showed no signs of being about to withdraw from the bliss of meditation, the scholar bowed his head thrice to the ground and softly departed. Within a year or so, he resigned from the Imperial Service and returned to his native township. There, having taken leave of his astonished wives and children, he repaired to a nearby monastery and enrolled as a simple novice. Step by step he rose to become a celebrated Dharma Master, who was eagerly sought after as a teacher of the liberating doctrine of Not Two.

4

Contemplative Practices

(a) INTRODUCTORY

In China, unlike in Japan, Tibet and elsewhere, the numerous Mahayana Buddhist sects long ago coalesced into a single form of Chinese Buddhism comprising six components: (i) observance by monks and nuns of the multifold *vinaya* rules of conduct and by laymen of the five precepts involving abstinence from killing, stealing, improper sexual intercourse, lying and the taking of intoxicants, coupled with the cultivation of compassion; (ii) rituals such as bowing down and making offerings to the Triple Gem, which are universal in all Buddhist countries; (iii) contemplative meditation combined with a minimal amount of philosophical study (inspired by the Ch'an (Zen) Sect); (iv) contemplative meditation based upon and supported by profound philosophical studies (largely inspired by the Hua Yen, T'ien T'ai and Wei Shih Sects); (v) contemplative meditation combined with the chanting of sacred formulas and invocation of the Celestial Buddhas and Bodhisattvas (inspired by the Ching T'u (Pure Land) Sect); (vi) some practices surviving from the days, more than a thousand years ago, when there was a Mi Tsung or Esoteric Sect which transmitted secret knowledge relating to the manipulation of powerful psychic forces with the assistance of mantras and mudrās, just like the teaching of Tibetan tantric masters today. This last sect disappeared after having incurred the particular hostility of the Confucian establishment, so that only fragments of its practices survive; whereas the contemplative sects very rarely suffered severe persecution. Broadly speaking, what are discussed in this section are practices relating to the third and fourth of the above categories.

(b) SUSTAINED AWARENESS

The practice of fixing sustained awareness upon bodily and mental processes, sequences of bodily movements, the rise and fall of emotions, or the immediate experience of Here and Now is very widespread in Buddhist countries, whether Theravadin or Mahayana. What to the uninstructed may at first seem a rather boring or even pointless exercise proves, upon experience, to be exceedingly worthwhile; for it is a prime means of diminishing ego-delusion; of transmuting negative emotions or causing them to subside; and of coming to recognise the true nature of being, in which will be discovered the identity of self and other. Though the exercises take numerous forms, the underlying purpose is to attain heightened insight into the nature of being, to which sustained awareness gives rise in a manner easier to experience than to explain. It is as though sustained awareness opens a door to unsuspected facets of the mystery of being. Some of the principal forms of practice are as follows:

Sitting in meditation posture, one directs attention to a selected part of the body, noting sensations usually too slight to be present to the consciousness and seeking to become more fully aware of what is going on there. Most often what one seeks to raise to the level of full consciousness is the entire breathing process, but the pulsing of the blood and indications of the functioning of the digestive process also have their importance in revealing how small a part in these processes is played by the supposed 'I'. Sometimes one experiments with different types of breathing, thinking: 'Now I am breathing in (or out) a short (medium or long) breath', and so on. Another variation is to attend to whatever mood, feeling or sensation is uppermost at the moment and concentrate on it, thinking: 'Now I will breathe in (or out) experiencing serenity (or whatever the uppermost sensation may be).' The combination of awareness and of conscious breathing seems to be particularly effective in leading to intuitive insight into the nature of being.[1] Again, one may direct attention to the mind, so as to observe successive thoughts or emotions with complete detachment, as though sitting back and watching them on a cinema screen. This, too, leads effectively to increasing insight into the absence of any entity that can properly be called 'I'.

While walking about (whether around a meditation hut or along a garden path specially for the purpose of cultivating awareness, or during an expedition to a market-place or other destination in connection with one's daily affairs), one concentrates attention on the sequences of bodily movement, thinking: 'Now I am raising my foot (lowering it, swinging my arm forward or backward, etc.).' This

[1] For a fuller account, see Lama Govinda's *Foundations of Tibetan Mysticism*, pp. 150–2.

exercise is performed for the same purpose as the sitting exercise just described. Getting into the habit of sustained awareness, no matter what one may happen to be doing, while adopting the attitude of an impartial observer, is highly effective yogically.

While engaged in daily affairs, dispassionate observation of what is happening within oneself, especially with regard to emotional states and their physical and psychological effects, is an admirable way of weakening the hold of passions or transmuting them into more wholesome states of mind. One reflects: 'Now anger (calm, joy, disappointment, envy) has arisen in my mind. Now my heart is beginning to beat faster (slower). Now my breath is coming in short gasps (growing more tranquil, etc.). Now I am experiencing an unpleasant secretion in my stomach (due to anger, fear, etc.). Now my face is growing red (pallid, etc.). Now I am stupidly giving way to an emotion that will surely result in harm to myself and others (or wisely refraining from . . . , etc.).' Such reflections, oft repeated and sustained, are bound to decrease the frequency of passionate conduct of a kind that will be bitterly regretted; they thus ensure increasing self-control.

While sitting or walking about, one concentrates one's awareness on details of the environment that normally escape notice, thinking: 'Now a ray of sunlight is illuminating those leaves. Now the bamboos are rustling in the wind, etc., etc.' This practice, besides opening the eyes to a thousand beauties commonly unnoticed or ignored, stimulates awareness of what may, in a sense, be called 'the only reality', since the past is no more than a memory, the future as yet a dream. The fuller one's awareness of the environment, the more immediate will become the sense of not being apart from it, of its constituting a very real extension of what one has formerly looked upon as a separate self.

The practice of awareness is valuable in many ways. Awareness of bodily and mental processes weakens the hold of ego-delusion, as one becomes increasingly aware of the extent to which actions, sensations, feelings, thoughts, emotions, etc., function or rise and wane without the intervention of anything in the nature of an ego. The once almighty 'I' is found to be very far from in command of a great many situations. When negative emotions such as anger arise, by maintaining the stance of a detached observer and noting the ugliness of their effects, one discovers how paltry, unwise or undesirable they are, and accordingly brings stillness of mind to bear on counteracting them. Awareness of the environment around one reveals the immediacy of Here and Now and helps the mind to withdraw from its ceaseless concern with ego-centred thoughts of past and future. Many people have become so much the slaves of remorse, expectation, anxiety and the idiotic play of jumbled thoughts as almost to have forgotten how to live in and enjoy the present. Friends who have driven a long distance to visit a famous park or lake or mountain scarcely give themselves time for a few rapturous exclamations before reverting to an endless dialogue about who has divorced or will soon divorce whom, whether such and such a merger will take place in Paris or Chicago, whether Miss X is likely to succumb to designs on her chastity, or who said what about which to whom. While all this nonsense is going on, the lovely lake sparkles unseen and the mountain which raises its lofty snowcapped head to a dazzlingly blue sky is ignored. In such trivialities perhaps as much as ninety per cent of their waking life is spent, for when they have no one to talk to, the endless colloquy goes on and on in their minds. So lacking in stillness are they that the sublime Tao, the Buddha Nature ever ready to shine around and within them, is totally obscured by dense clouds of inanity. Ah, what a waste of precious moments! Even a little training in sustained aware-ness would make a world of difference to their happiness and spare those around them from having to be ready with polite responses.

(c) CHIH KUAN

Influenced by the teachings of the T'ien T'ai Sect, many Chinese meditation teachers advocate strict adherence to a practice known as *chih kuan* which, in one form or another, is well nigh universal among the lamas who transmit the various Tibetan traditions. It consists of alternating two main types of meditation and should be practised throughout all but the most exalted stages of the Way. *Chih* (literally, 'stopping') and *kuan* (meaning 'discriminating contemplation') are necessary complements to each other.

Chih broadly covers all those kinds of meditation that aim at rising above conceptual thought, transcending normal states of conscious-ness, achieving inner stillness and opening the mind to the inflow of intuitive wisdom, in the light of which the real nature of all beings and of the entire cosmos is revealed. *Chih* meditation thus includes attaining one-pointedness of mind, as well as the state known as objectless awareness during which the consciousness resembles a bright lantern shining upon a limitless expanse of snow; contemplat-ing the embodiments of the energy of wisdom-compassion such as, for example, Kuan Yin Bodhisattva; and attaining *samadhi* by the use of invocations or mantras. It is by such means that the mystic achieves profound intuition of the true face of reality in its undifferentiated form. In its proper context, *chih* leads directly towards Enlightenment. Yet, if practised uninterruptedly during the whole course of every meditation session and resorted to whenever opportunities arise to withdraw the mind from its surroundings, it is attended by two great dangers; either the adept may 'get lost in the void' or draw back from it in terror. Of these, the first means that, clinging to the bliss of emptiness, he mistakes this experience for direct perception of the true face of reality, and may henceforth despise, dislike, or doubt the real existence of, the world like those Indian sages who speak of it as *maya* – pure delusion – and deny its reality. Supposing a mere stage of intuitive perception to be the final goal, he halts by the wayside and progresses no further; on this account, the treasure he set out to find is never gained! Lost in rapturous contemplation for hours together and feeling sadly exiled from that rapture when otherwise engaged, he becomes like a ghost in the eyes of others, whom he, in his turn, sees as ghosts. Far, far worse is the second danger; perception of the illimitable void may so terrify the adept that he halts upon the Way like a long-distance runner who stops short, screaming at the edge of a dark abyss. No-*thing*-ness suddenly appears to him as nothingness. I have said 'far, far worse' and yet, yogically, mistaking rapturous bliss for the goal is as great an error as falling to abject terror; in either case, progress is halted.

Kuan or discursive, discriminating contemplation involves, at least in the early and median stages, deliberate use of conceptual thought and resort to logic. Armed with some foreknowledge of the nature of the goal by his teachers, or from his own reading of, say, the incomparable works of Nagarjuna, the adept employs his learning to destroy dialectically false concepts such as the reality of ego-entities and the validity of the distinction between self and other, or the belief that beings and objects possess more than transient, wave-like individualities. By analytical observation of the functioning of his body and mind or of the I-less nature of their composition, and by intellectual deduction, he comes to realise, first conceptually and later intuitively, the unreality of self and of any kind of own-being. This requires thoughtful study of certain Mahayana doctrines as a support to meditation. In the absence of *chih*, however, *kuan* will not take him by any means all the way to his goal. To apprehend intellectually the void aspect of reality is not enough; and *kuan* will not enable him to realise it intuitively, unless supported by *chih*. Therefore the two practices should be alternated, whether several times during each relatively long meditation session – which is the way most commonly recommended – or by devoting alternate shorter sessions to each.

Chih is practised, usually in the meditation posture, by fixing the awareness so as to restrain the mind from wandering; thoughts as they arise are quietly abandoned, whereat blissful abstraction may supervene. *Kuan* is also generally practised while seated in the meditation posture and often follows immediately upon *chih*; most often it takes the form of reflecting analytically upon some specific aspect of the Buddha's teaching, such as the three characteristics of all compounded 'entities' – unsatisfactoriness, impermanence and absence of own-being; or on the impermanence, interdependence and (in an ultimate but not in a proximate sense) unreality of individual beings and objects; or on the impossibility of isolating an ego-entity from among the components of one's body-mind. Such reflection often requires calling to mind and pondering the arguments formulated by sages who have attained Enlightenment and propounded them as a means of leading pupils in the direction of the goal. Learning rather than intuition is employed in the early stages; later they are combined and, finally, pure intuition supervenes – but not without the aid of *chih*.

The adept does not need to work to a timetable in alternating the two practices. *Chih* is especially indicated when the mind is turbulent, when the attention wanders easily and idle thoughts grow clamorous; whereas *kuan* is required when the mind is torpid and unable to function effectively as a bright light shining upon undifferentiated infinity. The main thing is to approach each meditation session well prepared, by deciding in advance upon a particular *chih*- and a particular *kuan*-type meditation, so as to be able to pass smoothly from the one to the other and back again without having to stop and consider what next to do.

At an advanced stage, *kuan* becomes increasingly intuitive and ultimately *chih* and *kuan* merge; with the growth of wisdom, the use of conceptual thought during meditation is finally transcended, together with the dualism of form and void; the dual aspects of reality are revealed as Not Two. Beyond this, all is silence. The unenlightened cannot speak of what they have yet to experience; the enlightened have discovered that to convey their experience to those who have not shared it is as impossible as to convey a precise notion of colour and perspective to people blind from birth. Lao-tzû's dictum, 'He who knows does not speak; he who speaks does not know', is entirely pertinent to the final stages of the Way. Thenceforward only negatives and paradox will serve.

Among Ch'an (Zen) followers in the West, there are some who decry the need for learning in their eagerness to emphasise that Ch'an is 'a wordless' doctrine – despite the millions of words that have been written about it in recent years! This error may be due to their having taken certain sayings of the more iconoclastic Ch'an masters *out of their original context*, mistaking teaching given in particular circumstances for a universal rule. Personally, I have yet to meet a Chinese or Tibetan meditation teacher of *any* sect who does not insist on sound knowledge of the Mahayana doctrines as a necessary prerequisite for attainment of the goal; though they do also teach that, prior to Enlightenment, there comes a stage at which all doctrines and set practices can be discarded.

Of the practices taught in this book, those set forth in II, B, 2, (e) and (f), and II, B, 4, (d) pertain largely or wholly to *chih*; those set forth in II, B, 4, (e), (f) and (g) pertain to *kuan*.

(d)   CH'AN (ZEN) MEDITATION

There used to be in China, as in Japan today, several schools of Ch'an Buddhism, all with specially favoured contemplative techniques. The principal aim, however, has always been to arrive through *chih*-type meditation at direct perception of one's true nature, which turns out to be not a personal possession, but identical with the nature of cosmic being. To speak of *one's own* true nature would be inapposite, and so the Chinese words for 'own nature' are not used in this context, the correct terms being *pên hsing* (original nature), *pên hsin* (original heart/mind) and *Fu Hsing* (the Buddha Nature), all three of which are recognised by the enlightened mind to be one and the same. In order to achieve direct perception of his original nature, the meditator seeks to attain a state of mind that is unsullied by the arising of a single thought and yet marvellously alert – the very antithesis of blank or torpid. Meanwhile, all objects to which the unenlightened mind tends to cling, such as appearances, names, terms, views, etc., must be discarded.

It may come as a surprise to Westerners to learn that the Japanese Rinzai *koan* technique, which has achieved such fame in recent decades, is not – and may never have been – current in its present form among Chinese Buddhists, for all that the *koans* themselves are of Chinese origin, being called *kung an* in that language. The long series of *kung an* (*koans* or paradoxical conundrums) with which Rinzai meditators are expected to wrestle one after another are pithy accounts of enigmatic episodes that originated in particular sets of circumstances and vary for that reason; all without exception reflect the same truth and, properly employed, lead to the same awakened state of mind; so the Chinese hold that there is no advantage to be gained from treating them, out of context, as a series leading progressively from elementary to profound.

The Chinese technique is to employ just one brief conundrum (known technically as a *hua t'ou*) and stick to that for as long as anything of the kind remains necessary, though a meditator is free to change over to another if, after diligent practice, he fails to make headway with the one originally assigned. As pointed out by Master Hsü Yün, the most revered Ch'an master of this century, and brought to the attention of Western readers by Lu K'uan Yü (Charles Luk) in his *Secrets of Chinese Meditation*, each *hua t'ou* contains or implies the key-word 'who?', for example 'Who is reverencing the Buddha?' or 'Before my parents were born, what was my original face [= who was I]?' One repeatedly propounds this conundrum to oneself, both during meditation sessions and at other times as well, for the practice should continue with hardly any interruption all day long, whether one is walking, standing, sitting or lying. The meditator does not seek a verbal answer, nor one dictated by logic or conceptual thought, for the intention is to halt the arising of thoughts in the mind. Besides, before embarking on the practice, he is likely to know already that, insofar as the answer can be conveyed in words, it is 'Mind' – not 'my mind', 'his mind', but just 'Mind' in the sense of 'The One Mind' that is the source, the non-substance and the goal of all being. The answer he seeks now is something not to be named or merely known, but *directly experienced* through an awakening to the nature of original Mind.

The *hua t'ou* is in the form of a question so that it may give rise to a doubt. Hitherto, one has taken it for granted that 'I am I' without seeking to discover just what this I-entity may be. With the help of Nagarjuna's admirable dialectics, one may attain to intellectual understanding of the fact that a close examination of the constituents of an individual's body-mind reveals no entity that can properly be called the ego; but Nagarjuna set no store by intellectual understanding of this fact, except as a preliminary guide leading towards intuitive experience. Intellectual processes, though exceedingly useful at the time of entering upon the Way and traversing its earlier stages, have sooner or later to be abandoned. One has to delve deeply into the mind and transcend conceptual thought in order to attain to direct experiential perception of that which lies behind the mere appearance of an 'I', namely vast, eternal, undifferentiated Mind.

The *hua t'ou*, though an effective means to the end in view, is itself impure, being a thought that sullies the absolute purity of a mind freed from *all* thought. It functions like the tiny hole left in a flask so that the air can be sucked out in order to create a perfect vacuum, after which the hole is sealed, that is to say the *hua t'ou* is abandoned. During practice, the chosen *hua t'ou* must not be pursued with ferocious energy or grim determination – quite the contrary. Whether sitting in meditation, strolling about or dealing with the necessary business of living, the meditator tries never to lose sight of his *hua t'ou* and keeps it as close as possible to the centre of his awareness at all times; all other thoughts are either totally excluded or, when the business of carrying on living absolutely demands their entry for a little while, relegated to the mind's periphery. Yet the *hua t'ou* must be dealt with so tranquilly that it barely causes a ripple in the otherwise undisturbed stillness; if it is pursued with frantic intensity on the one hand or carelessly and infrequently on the other, the answer will never dawn in the consciousness and the whole exercise will be wasted. Awareness is concentrated on this one thought with calm persistence: 'Who is reverencing the Buddha – who–o–o–o–o–o?' Causing, as it does, sustained doubt as to the validity of ordinary experience, the conundrum insistently stirs the mind which, emptied of all other thought, draws closer and closer to the sudden awakening that brings the meditator face to face with his original nature – the Buddha Nature, undifferentiated void, the Tao!

This use of the phrase 'sudden awakening' may recall the famous controversy between exponents of the Northern and Southern Schools of Ch'an, with the former claiming that the awakening is gradual, the latter asserting that it is sudden. Both, of course, were right. Awakening is gradual in that a long-drawn-out process is involved, as when a tea-kettle filled with cold water is gradually brought to the boil over a small charcoal stove. It is sudden in that, instead of beginning to dawn at an early stage and gradually intensifying, it occurs abruptly, as when the water in the kettle, having long been rising in temperature without any other notable change occurring, suddenly reaches boiling-point and bubbles fiercely, rattling the kettle's lid.

As to the term 'awakening', the Japanese word for it, *satori*, may cause confusion in the minds of Western readers – my own, for one. In English-language books about Zen, the epithets 'major' and 'minor' are sometimes applied to *satori*. Now, the Chinese equivalent of *satori* is *chieh wu*, meaning 'awakening' in the sense of Enlightenment, which is not something that can be experienced by degrees. I take it, then, that *satori* is a word used in Japan to cover a whole range of intuitive experiences *leading in the direction of* Enlightenment, as well as Enlightenment itself. If so, one must be careful to avoid the error of supposing that the first faint flash of intuition is identical in intensity with what is known to all Buddhists as Unexcelled Enlightenment. The point needs to be made because, in the West where Buddhism is still in its infancy, one occasionally comes across people who claim to have attained Enlightenment, though without exhibiting any of the signs that attend that exalted state. I am convinced that a truly enlightened person would never under any circumstances make that claim for himself; for, with Enlightenment, the last trace of egocentricity vanishes, leading to the perception that *there is no individual to be Enlightened*, whereas the assertion 'I am Enlightened' implies the contrary. Besides, one of the outstanding qualities by which true sages can be recognised is an endearing *modesty*.

A person new to the practice of Ch'an meditation should start with one, two or three quite short periods of sitting each day, preferably at regular times, and gradually lengthen the sessions until they are as long as he can manage without putting too much strain on himself or experiencing a feeling of staleness. In the intervals between sessions, he should return frequently to contemplation of his *hua t'ou*, but not push himself too hard, as to do so is not helpful and may even result in a nervous breakdown. There should be reasonable exertion, as when an athlete in training pushes himself every few days to do just a little more than he can very comfortably do at each successive stage of training, but no forcing of the issue, no tightly clenched teeth, no fierce Samurai spirit of do or die! The Buddha's teaching is known as the Middle Path; all kinds of extremes are to be avoided.

Like most people trained by Chinese masters (among whom, however, there are *some* exceptions), I do not believe that maintaining the lotus posture at the cost of severe leg pains is advisable. Pain can scarcely be good in itself, since it inevitably distracts the mind from contemplation of the *hua t'ou* – though just a little pain, incurred as the sessions are gradually prolonged by a few minutes every few days, does no harm. I wonder if those meditators who advocate enduring prolonged pain as a useful discipline are aware that the lotus posture was evolved at a time when Asians were so accustomed to sitting on the floor or cross-legged on a couch that they found sitting in a chair positively uncomfortable? In fact, the lotus posture was lauded by the sages of old as the *most comfortable* way of sitting still for several hours at a time. Personally, I recommend a practice I observed among the Zen community at Tassajara, California, where the small cushion sometimes placed upon a large, square meditation cushion to accommodate the buttocks, and thereby reduce pressure on the legs, was made higher than those normally used by Asians, as if to compensate for the differences between Asian and Caucasian build. Ability to endure pain uncomplainingly, though an asset in some circumstances, does not strike me as being in the least conducive to successful meditation.

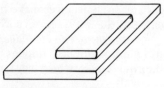 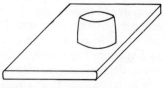

Traditional-style cushions   Adapted upper cushion

Summary – Some elementary rules

(i) Do not sit very long at a time, initially. Lengthen the sessions gradually and not too ambitiously. Try to adhere to regular times, morning and evening, every day; and do not miss out a session, if that can be avoided.

(ii) Attempt the lotus posture at every session, but revert to sitting cross-legged tailor-fashion rather than endure distracting leg pain. Support the buttocks with a relatively high cushion, if necessary to reduce pain.

(iii) Remember that working on a single *hua t'ou*, as long as it gives rise to the necessary state of doubt, can be quite as effective as a progressive series of *koans*.

(iv) It may be found more effective to use the Chinese form of the *hua t'ou* – *Nien Fu shih shei?* (literally, 'Reverencing the Buddha is who?') – as, besides being shorter, it has the advantage of ending emphatically with the key-word '*who–o–o*'. The word *shih* is quite similar to the word 'sure' when pronounced by Americans in a manner that, to my Englishman's ear, sounds very much like 'shrrrr'.

(v) Be gently persistent in making the *hua t'ou* the centre of sustained awareness, but modelling your practice on water invisibly eroding a stone, not on a gale uprooting a tree. Avoid rigidity, tension, strain.

(iv) Commence and terminate each session with three prostrations to the Buddha, as a remedy for the dangerous spiritual pride that may otherwise attend increasing success. It is by reverence and awe for the greater-than-self that egotistic feelings are subdued.

(e) CONTEMPLATION OF NO SELF

This is a *kuan*-type or discursive meditation, which begins at the level of conceptual thought and seems at first to be only an intellectual approximation of the subtle insights into the nature of reality gained through pure intuition; yet so closely does it touch upon what becomes apparent during *chih*-type meditation that its practice will in time lead beyond conceptual thought into the realm of direct intuitive experience, especially if it is alternated with the one-pointed concentration described in the concluding paragraph. My account of it is based upon a contemplative work by the Fifth Dalai Lama, recently translated by Geshe Rabden and Geoffrey Hopkins. If in simplifying it I have transgressed by departing from its essence in any way, the fault must be ascribed to me, not to the exalted author or learned translators.

Having taken up the meditation posture, the adept reminds himself that beings and objects are identical in nature with the undifferentiated non-substance of the void, of which all seeming entities are but transient manifestations. To hold that the ego or self is an independent entity is to deny the voidness of its nature and to suppose that it exists independently of all other manifestations of the void, which is also the One Mind. To accept that the ego is not real is to recognise its intrinsic voidness and its total interdependence on all manifestations of the void, and especially to conclude that no such thing as an ego principle can be isolated from the five constituents of being (*skandhas*) that together compose a person's body-mind.

The first step is known as 'ascertaining the object to be negated'. The adept conceives of his 'self' as though it really did exist, and recalls some of the occasions on which this 'I' has been made to suffer or rejoice by the words or actions of other people. He tries to note exactly what he takes this 'I' to be, for example what is its relationship to the rest of his body, mind, feelings and discriminations, and what are the constituents of which he deems it to be composed. He may perhaps reflect: 'I, Peter Jones, am undoubtedly a real person. I recall how upset I was when my sister called me a good-for-nothing in front of a lot of people, and how I enjoyed the critical acclaim that greeted my recent novel. By "I", I mean this person seated here, an individual mind contained in an individual body, now enjoying the warmth of the sun and remembering how unpleasant it is to feel really cold. This "I" is clearly related to my mind, since it can be hurt by disparagement and elated by praise; but also to my body, since it responds to warmth and shrinks from cold.'

The second step, known as 'ascertaining pervasion', is to reflect that the 'I' must either be one with or else separate from the five aggregates of personality – namely *form* (body, sense organs, etc.), *feelings* (both physical and mental, including pleasant, unpleasant and neutral), *perceptions* (of colour, smell, taste, etc., as well as the ability to recognise, discriminate, identify), *conditionings* (including volitions, responses, reactions such as pride or fear, impulses, tendencies, judgements and 'movements of the mind to objects' as when one reflects that something is desirable or otherwise) and *consciousness* (awareness of things implying a separation of subject and object, and awareness of the other aggregates listed above). Logically the 'I' has to be either the same, or not the same, as these five. One may perhaps reflect:

'If "I" is not something apart from these five aggregates, why do I tend to speak of "*my* body, *my* perceptions", etc.? Surely that is tantamount to saying "my I" or "body's body"? How absurd that would sound! Very well, then, I must suppose that "I" means just my mind. Yet how can that be? Can mind feel cold or hunger, or require to be fed and clothed? Certainly not, but "I" does feel and require those things, so it seems more likely that "I" comprises all five of those aggregates including form [the body]. But, in that case, either there must be five different "I"s, or else the five aggregates are really one – neither of which makes sense. Nor does it make the least sense to say that "I" is neither different from, nor the same as, the five aggregates.'

The third step is called 'ascertaining the lack of true identity between the self and the five aggregates of personality'. One recognises that the 'I' must be different from those five, since each of them can be clearly recognised for what it is, whereas it appears that the "I" cannot be thus identified. He may reflect:

'So "I" is different from those five? Yet, though I can identify my body by touch, feel things as pleasant or otherwise, discriminate between red and green, note my tendency to enjoy working with my brain but not with my hands, and be conscious of that clump of trees over there as an object of my mind, I can by no means touch, feel, discriminate, enjoy or be conscious of as an object of my mind an entity apart from these five that is identifiable as "I". In short, "I" is just an empty concept having no recognisable validity at all.' Meditating thus, day after day, with unlimited variations, the adept is bound to reach this same conclusion again and again. Increasingly he will become convinced that 'I' and 'mine' are no more than conventional terms to disguise a fiction for the sake of day-to-day convenience. This recognition, when it moves from the intellectual level and becomes a matter of direct intuitive perception, brings liberation – Enlightenment!

During each session, after engaging in variations of this analysis of the so-called 'I', the adept should switch over to a form of *chih*-practice based on the same theme, by concentrating one-pointedly on a single object which, when the mind has been still for a little while, should be replaced by the thought ' "I" has no inherent existence'. This thought now becomes the object of one-pointed concentration. An alternative practice is to go forwards and backwards several times within a single session between the *kuan*-type analysis aimed at negating the 'I'-concept and the *chih*-type one-pointed concentration just mentioned. This two-pronged attack will inevitably result in the diminution and final disappearance of ego-based delusion.

(f)   IDENTIFICATION OF SELF AND OTHER

This meditation is not essentially different in aim from the previous one. The adept commences by carrying out a similar *kuan*-type analysis of the constituents of an object chosen at random – let it be, in this instance, a dark-red four-legged wooden stool – and seeks to identify it as an independently existing object possessing something in the nature of own-being. Mentally removing the legs and placing them beside the flat seat, he recognises that it is no longer a stool, although all its parts are present. Contemplating its colour, he reflects that this depends not only on the quality of light and shade, but also on the eye of the beholder, since there are some people who perceive red as green, some who deem dark red beautiful and others who intensely dislike it. Noting what he conceived to be the shape of the stool before it was dismantled, he observes that this, too, was a mirage, since the 'shape' of an object depends upon the angle from which it is viewed; and he recollects that any given object is at once both large and small, as the concept of size depends upon what is taken as the basis of comparison. Reflecting on the material of which it is composed, he remarks that the wood came from a certain tree that would not have been the same tree, nor have grown exactly where it did, had not its remote ancestors survived forest fires and pestilences over a period of ten million years and more. Thus he comes to see that his chosen object is utterly devoid of the quality of individual, independent being. It has no intrinsic quality that could be described as 'essence of stool-ness'. In fact, it was only a stool for as long as its components stood in a certain relation to one another and, even then, it might have been taken for a table by people of another culture and thus *become* a table without the slightest alteration of its form. The stool, then, is not necessarily a stool; its colour, shape and size depend upon innumerable factors, including the viewers (who themselves are the products of infinitely long and varied chains of causes and effects); the material of which it is composed is the fruit of things that have happened and not happened since before the coming into being of the universe.

With these observations as a starting-point, he reflects: 'Nothing possesses a nature that can properly be called its own, since each transient manifestation of the void depends upon an infinitude of preceding and concurrent causes stretching back to the beginningless beginning, forward to eternity and outward to the furthest galaxy. So, too, myself. Everything within the vast cosmic environment, including that puny object I have hitherto thought much of, taking it to be "myself", is quite literally dependent on everything else. All are transient, interdependent manifestations of the void. Since I and others are identical in nature and have nothing we can truly call our, own except for what belongs equally to all, how foolish is the pride I have hitherto taken in my so-called "unique individuality"! Just as I have lived my life forever striving to keep at bay dissatisfaction, suffering, premature decay and dissolution, so must it be with every living thing, whether god, man, elephant, ant, demon, tree, flower, vegetable or weed! Perceiving the identical nature of all beings and objects throughout the limitless cosmos, I accept that every one of them is as close to me as bone of my bone, flesh of my flesh. Aware that my endeavours to win a full measure of health, well-being and longevity are shared by every sentient being, how dare I make much of myself or belittle others?

'Since nature decrees that nourishment is needed to sustain life, I am bound to eat and thus compelled to acquiesce in the destruction of living things; indeed, I cannot inhale a single breath, drink a glass of spring water, set foot upon the ground, turn over in my sleep or use the mildest of medicines without the risk of inadvertently destroying numberless sentient beings. Nevertheless, in the light of my heightened understanding, I shall refrain from deliberate intrusion upon (and do my utmost to promote) the welfare and happiness of all people, animals and plants. My slavish concern for myself at the expense of other beings has been ignoble; henceforth I shall cultivate compassion and sympathetic understanding towards all that live. Never again must I permit myself to do wilful harm to the least regarded of the myriad beings. Life is sacred because the life of one is the life of all. Even that fine though hitherto unattainable concept, the brotherhood of man, is a paltry matter in relation to the kinship of all beings within the universe. If there are galaxies removed from ours by a million light-years, the creatures that may dwell there are to some extent dependent on me, and I on them. May I never again relapse into the folly of ego-centredness!'

Meditation along these lines, accompanied by a firm intention to act in the light of the insights gained, will sweep away many obstacles from the path to Enlightenment.

(g) HUA YEN MEDITATION

The Hua Yen Ching (Gaṇḍavyūha Avataṁsaka Sūtra) is a mind-boggling work, as readers familiar with the excerpts from it contained in Garma Chang's *The Buddhist Teaching of Totality* know well. The most profound of the sutras, it proclaims an exalted doctrine that transcends the furthest reaches of ordinary logic in a manner so persuasive that one staggers back, mind reeling, from the contemplation of literally billions of universes all interpenetrating one another. In China, this sutra became the basis of a sublime system of meditation from which the simplified practices described below derive. Some premises of Hua Yen philosophy are: All things originate in total dependence on all others and are devoid of selfhood; consequently, only void can properly be said to exist; yet there is no void apart from tangible phenomena; non-being coexists with being, no separation being possible. The myriad manifestations comprising the 'all' are empty in substance and thus identical in nature with the 'one'. What is more, *the small contains the great* no less than the great contains the small; indeed, *entities penetrate into and contain one another without the slightest hindrance*, each being at once a reflection and reflector of all others.

The vast implications of the italicised words cannot be satisfactorily indicated in a few paragraphs. Interested readers are referred to Dr Chang's extraordinary book. Here we are concerned with the practical use that can be made of these concepts as a basis for some relatively simple meditations.

An idea of the underlying philosophy can be gained from an

account given in that book of a demonstration arranged by Dharma Master Fa Tsang for the Empress Wu Tsê-t'ien (reigned AD 684 – 705). The Master prepared a hall by covering ceiling, floor, walls and the four corners with huge mirrors facing one another; in the centre was a Buddha image with a burning torch beside it. Every mirror reflected not only the actual Buddha image and the reflections of it contained in the other mirrors, but also the reflections of reflections of reflections of these reflections to an extent approximating to infinity. Then he produced a crystal ball, within the small circumference of which the Empress saw an infinitude of Buddha images. Thus did the Dharma Master demonstrate by a kind of visual analogy that the small contains the great, and that countless entities can penetrate one another without obstruction.

The following meditations were suggested by some of the much more complicated ones devised by the first and a later patriarch of the Hua Yen Sect, namely Master Tu Shun (AD 558 – 640) and Master Fa Tsang (643–712).

(i)   *Meditation on true voidness*

The purpose is to demolish the erroneous view that true voidness exists apart from form. Although the realm of form reported by our senses has many deceptive characteristics, there is no absolute void lying outside or in any way apart from this tangible realm.

The meditator, seated in the open or gazing through a window (it might be the window of an aeroplane), contemplates the clouds on one of those days when they are plentiful and undergoing rather swift transformations. He reflects: 'Those mountains, seas, islands, peninsulas and castles in the sky are formed of one substance, cloud; all are identical in nature. This provides an analogy with the uniformly void nature of all objects in the universe and illustrates the doctrine "form is void"; for, just as there is no abstract cloud lying apart from its tangible shifting forms, so is there no void apart from form – void *is* form! These two are one; the difference depends upon whether form or substance lies uppermost in our awareness.' Watching the clouds undergoing their everlasting changes, he builds a series of detailed analogies to illustrate the principle thus enunciated – perhaps for half an hour or so.

He then turns his attention to the tallest feature in his surroundings and reflects: 'To suppose that there are other and taller hills behind the one at which I am gazing would be pure speculation unjustified by anything within the scope of my knowledge, whereas that hill is a fact of experience. So, too, would it be speculative and unjustified to suppose that there is an absolute realm of void lying apart from the objects of perception whose reality I experience. Where I may go wrong is not in denying a reality behind reality (since there is nothing of the sort), but in concluding that hand or eye can reveal the true nature of what I touch and see. These things are not real just because I touch and see them, my perceptions of them being necessarily faulty; their reality derives from their true nature – which is void. In other words, the trees and hills around me are not opaque ghosts, dark visions or delusions hiding something that lies beyond; delusion lies in supposing them to be as permanent as they look and to possess individual own-nature. That even rocks are not permanent is a matter of common knowledge. That things possess no true individuality becomes obvious when one looks in vain for any entity within them that could properly be described as own-being, and when one realises that they could not have come even into temporary existence in the absence of a myriad chains of cause and effect inextricably linking them to everything else within the universe. Take this tree or rock, for instance. That it is devoid of own-being, in the sense of some inherent tree-ness or hill-ness, can be demonstrated by mentally reducing it to a heap of sawdust or mound of fine powder from which not one grain of the original mass has been removed; though its constituent parts are all present, it is no longer a tree or rock. To understand that it could not exist in the absence of everything else, I must reflect upon some of the happenings that brought them into transient existence – happenings depending on happenings depending on happenings forever widening in their circumference, extending backward to infinity, outwards to the furthest corners of the universe. Form, then, is void. This tree or rock, possessing no intrinsic own-being or apartness from everything else, is like one of those cloud formations that change in a few moments from the likeness of an old man's face to that of a castle or a dragon, except for the trifling circumstance that the time-scale of *visible* change is different. Void, then, is form. It does not exist apart from trees, hills and all the rest. Voidness is the universal non-substance, yet inseparable from forms.'

Up to this point, the meditation has been largely an intellectual exercise. Although some degree of intuition may already have dawned during the course of it, it has been primarily a kind of drill intended to foster intellectual understanding in preparation for what follows. Now the meditator, abandoning all concepts, concentrates his mind one-pointedly on an object of his choice and, having attained to stillness, substitutes for that object the single thought 'No own-being' – not to be dwelt upon discursively, but merely taken as the focus of awareness. If he wishes, he may repeat the words over and over like a mantra.

These *kuan*- and *chih*-type practices can be alternated several times within a single session. Without *kuan* to build up some preliminary understanding, *chih* might prove unavailing; yet, when *chih* is actually being performed, intellectual understanding must not be allowed to clutter the mind. In course of time, intuitive insight is likely to flow abundantly from the alternation of these two.

(ii)   *Meditation on 'The small contains the great'*

This concept should not strike thoughtful Westerners as bizarre. Both Tennyson and Emerson arrived at the perception that a tiny object, such as a flower or grain of sand, embraces the entire universe. The English philosopher Whitehead's *Philosophy of Organism* sheds some light upon this concept, as does the work of Master Tu Shun. Unfortunately, the patriarch's instructions for meditation, contained in his *Meditation on the All-Embracing Totality*, are far from simple. Nevertheless, his teaching that each atom of the universe can, without expansion, embrace innumerable universes is so important that I have ventured to construct a more simple meditation which I believe will be effective; the outline came to me after reading Garma Chang's rendering of Master Fa Tsang's treatise entitled *On the Golden Lion*. In that work, the statue of a lion standing outside the Empress Wu's palace symbolises the realm of form; the solid gold of which it was made symbolises the void non-substance of the universe. He explains that all the various parts of the lion take in the whole in that all alike are pure gold. Thus, for example, every one of them permeates the lion's eyes, which are therefore also the ears, the nose, etc. Equally, every part of it, down to each single hair, contains the whole lion, together with all the innumerable lions embraced by its tiny parts. (The obvious fallacy in this argument arises from the fact that gold, being a solid substance, is subject to measurement and spatial laws; the fallacy no longer obtains when we translate 'gold' into measureless, non-spatial void.)

The meditation I derived from this runs as follows: The meditator takes some small object in his hand, say, a daisy. He reflects: 'Here is a flower. It is as real as can be, but its reality has nothing to do with transient characteristics such as its colour, shape, softness and so forth; it is real just because it manifests infinite being – the Tao. Yet, since infinite being is entirely devoid of characteristics, it would be nonsense to tell myself that I am holding a predominantly white and very small piece of infinity. The flower's colour and relative smallness are merely transient manifestations of that which has no colour and no size. The non-substance of the universe, like mind or consciousness, is not subject to measurement or the operation of spatial laws. One cannot have *a piece* of mind! If what I hold in my hand is identified as infinite being, then my hand is indeed grasping the entire universe! In contemplating this flower, I am contemplating no "drop in the ocean of infinite being", but the ocean of being in its entirety, since every drop possesses the quality of infinitude and is thus 'coextensive' with the whole.'

At this point, logic fails. To go further, one has to abandon conceptual thought and rely on the marvellous intuition that has enabled certain poets and philosophers to perceive the entire universe in every flower and grain of sand. The meditator now ceases to philosophise and concentrates his whole awareness upon the flower in his hand. Having attained to stillness, he transfers his awareness from the flower to the phrase 'infinite being'; whereupon, after a while, *samadhi* is likely to supervene. Presently, withdrawing from *samadhi* or from whatever approximate state of consciousness he has entered, he returns to discursive contemplation of the flower, then back to one-pointedness of mind and so on.

(iii) *Meditation on 'All entities penetrate and contain each other'*
One begins by recalling Master Fa Tsang's demonstration in the hall prepared for the Empress Wu, reflecting: 'That the crystal ball could contain a myriad Buddha images, many of them larger than itself, was due to their being reflections greatly reduced in size. At the level of ordinary everyday observation, it would not seem possible for a crystal ball of small dimensions to contain an infinitude of objects including some much larger than itself. However, the true nature of all objects is void, non-spatial. During a dream in which the dreamer beholds Mount Kanchenjunga, it can be said that this vast mountain and all the objects in the foreground exist within him. This is possible because, being non-spatial in character, the dreamer's mind has no bounds. But, according to sages versed in Mahayana teachings and enlightened by the direct perception bestowed by intuitive wisdom, the whole universe is a creation of Mind. Therefore everything whatsoever is a mental creation. The laws of space hold good at the level of appearances, but not at the level of reality, so there is no difficulty in understanding that all objects are containable within the small circumference of each one of them, just as Kanchenjunga fits comfortably into a dreamer's mind. There is, then, no hindrance whatever to their mutual penetration. Mount Kanchenjunga, being

essentially a mind creation, can contain the forms of dreamers as easily as dreamers can contain the forms of mountains within the tiny circumference of their skulls!'

Having got thus far by a logical process, the meditator now stills his mind by concentrating one-pointedly upon an object of his choice; then he transfers his one-pointed awareness to the mental image of a small crystal ball and views therein a multitude of objects – making no judgements, seeking no explanations, indulging in no mental inventory of what he sees, but just gazing at the mental image. By this means, he opens up his mind to the influx of intuitive wisdom; what started as make-believe may be revealed in the light of such wisdom as more intensely real than all the visible objects in his surroundings. As before, these *kuan* and *chih* practices should be alternated.

(h)   A STORY

A certain student at Tsinghua University during the 1940s, whom we shall call Sung, was the son of a Christian Chinese tin-mine owner in what was then called the Federation of Malaya; he had come to study in Peking largely in order to perfect his knowledge of literary Chinese. Rather to his own surprise, he soon began to take a deep interest in Buddhism. At weekends and during vacations, he would visit the dilapidated temples within the walls of the ancient capital, which had not recovered from the impoverishment that had befallen them during the long Japanese occupation recently ended, or go to stay at one or other of two important monasteries lying deep in the Western Hills. At first it had been their atmosphere of peace that had attracted him. When I asked if he had become a Buddhist, he explained that one thing held him back. 'I find it impossible', he said, 'to accept the unreality of my "self". I do realise that one's seeming to oneself to be the centre of the universe is sheer delusion, as everyone with the smallest intelligence must know. All the same, I can't help feeling that my "I" is a very real – and sometimes tiresome – entity. *I* want to eat or sleep, and so *I* dine or go to bed. *I* like staying in temples and learning about Buddhism, because *I* am keenly interested in *my own* intellectual and spiritual development. The Mahayana teachings have failed to convince me that the Imperious Master, as I call my ego, has no existence.'

At about this time (1947), Sung happened to meet a disciple of the famous Ch'an Master Hsü Yün, who, on coming to know the young man well, put the matter thus: 'When bodies are dissected and all their organs carefully studied by anatomists, no trace of an ego- or soul-repository is to be found – that goes without saying. Again, should a person involved in a serious accident have most of his limbs amputated, I think you will agree that what you call his ego would not be diminished thereby. So your ego, if it exists, must surely be located in your mind. Agreed?'

Sung nodded, having been fully persuaded of this since first becoming interested in the subject. 'Good, very good,' exclaimed the monk. 'Yet can something altogether formless and intangible be situated in something equally formless and intangible? I think not. When a cloud enters a cloud, they merge. Would not the same be true of such intangible entities as ego and mind? Your ego, then, can hardly reside *in* your mind, so it looks as though it must *be* your mind. Is that possible? Not long ago you told me you had felt impelled to visit the willow lanes (a district of courtesans) in the quarter of the city lying beyond Ch'ien Mên, on a night when you had intended to participate in celebrating Kuan Yin Bodhisattva's birthday at the Nien Hua Monastery. You added that you had given way to that somewhat undignified urge with reluctance amounting to sorrow. Is that not a case of body saying yes peremptorily in reply to mind's mournful no? Where was your ego in this? It seems to have aligned itself with your body in doing battle with your mind. If so, how can ego and mind be one?'

The monk, having followed this up with further examples to prove that the so-called ego is to be equated neither wholly with the body, nor wholly with the mind, nor yet with both of them or neither, continued: 'Would you not say, then, that one's whole being, one's whole body-mind is forever being pulled this way and that by numbers of conflicting forces to which a fool gives way without reflection, thus allowing them to make of him a poor, bedraggled shuttlecock; whereas the wise man learns to resist their push and pull? Just so.'

Unable to controvert this, Sung had nodded silently. Now the monk continued: 'The kind of men most admired over the centuries by thoughtful people living in this world of dust are those like the Enlightened One and, in the Western regions, Jesus of Nazareth – sages who won acclaim just on account of being the opposite of egocentric. They exemplify the spirit of victory – but victory over what? If you say a victory of mind over mind, you credit them with having two or three minds in one body. How can that be? Their victory, rather, was over those pushing and pulling forces. But if your ego lies in them, it is surprisingly extensive and includes all sorts of things outside your mind-body, such as gold, jade and pearls, mansions with elegantly lacquered beams and doorways, beautiful women with moth-like eyebrows and willowy gait. Do not the pushes and pulls derive from such as these? True, some components of those forces are karmic propensities inherited by your body-mind from past lives or generated by your thoughts and actions in the present life; yet they cannot be your ego, for with good training and Bodhisattva-like determination they can be eliminated. When they lose their push and pull, would you say that your ego then disappears? If so, it is a poor kind of thing, a mere bundle of appendages that can be tossed into a ditch.'

Sung stared at him uncomfortably and I – a silent witness to this interview – could not help smiling.

'Now,' said the monk, 'I shall tell you what it is that you have been mistaking for an inborn "I". Some of its components are situated in your body with its eight orifices and various sense organs – but flesh, blood, bone and skin change so fast that, after a few years, not a particle of what I see before me now will still be present. Some of its components are your feelings of pleasant and unpleasant, but these just come and go. When the child who greedily munches sweetmeats dripping with syrup and detests the stink of *ta-ch'iu* (grain spirit) becomes a man, his taste for honeyed sweetmeats will be gone, whereas he will down cup after cup of *ta-ch'iu* with the greatest enjoyment. Pleasant and unpleasant will have replaced each other! Part of what you take to be your ego comprises impulses, volitions, strivings and so forth – these, as you know, are capable of changing from hour to hour, if not minute to minute. Part is constituted by your bundle of perceptions, your discriminations between beautiful and ugly, desirable and loathsome, good and bad – need I say these also change? My uncle, a much-married man, used to rave about the beauty of one girl after another, but those he secured as minor wives lost all attraction for him within a month or so. A moon-faced beauty can scarcely become an overfed cow within the space of a few weeks, but such was the terminology that bore witness to the speed with which my uncle's perception of beauty changed! Another part of your ego-delusion is your consciousness which, being impure and deceived by your senses, insists upon a duality between "I" and "other". Yet that, too, can change within an hour or less, as when a meditator, on achieving a heightened state of consciousness, perceives all distinction between subject and object to be void, as may sometimes happen also, I am told, after inhaling more than the usual number of pipes of opium. I myself have never been much given to taking pleasure in women, opium or spirits. I dwell on these analogies because I am speaking of what is true for everyone, whether saints or profligates.

'Truly you are identifiable as a person with a name and form all your own, but the name Layman Sung is a mere convenience; it denotes no more than a fortuitous combination of five heaps or bundles (*skandhas*) that are perpetually involved in change. Not an atom of your body-mind remains unchanged through life. You may be recognisable from photographs taken of you at a tender age through a close similarity of form, but the constituents of that form have all been replaced since the photographs were taken. Your ego does not – cannot – reside in those five heaps, yet not a hair's tip of any part of you lies outside them. Where then is your ego? Ah, abandon this dangerous delusion, that your mind may be purified and become aware of its true holiness, its infinite vastness, its identity with Mind, with the Buddha-Nature!'

It would be satisfying to report that young Sung, awakened by these words of wisdom, progressed rapidly towards Enlightenment. As far as I could judge, he did not. Even so, the monk's eloquence (much more persuasive than I have been able to make it seem here, now that so many years have passed since I heard it) did convince him that the doctrine of 'no self' may well embody a correct interpretation of the real state of things. He no longer saw it as something to be rejected out of hand. Willingly he agreed to practice some meditations that the monk had recommended.

When I saw him last, a few days before both of us left Peking then on the point of being submerged by the red flood, he said: 'I doubt if I am very competent at meditation, for my old friend Ego still dictates a good deal of what I do and say and think. Still, there are signs that the old bandit will one day lose his grip. Quite often in my meditations there come moments when I find him gone!'

5

Compassion Yoga

(a) INTRODUCTORY

To perform this important and most promptly effective of the yogas
known to me personally, it is necessary to attend to three prerequis-
ites:

(i) One must be able to accept without reservation that, within
Mind and therefore latent in the minds of all, there exists in potential
form the transforming power known as *bodhi*, of which Buddha-like
wisdom and compassion are the twin constituents. Knowledge of its
existence has been arrived at intuitively by mystics of many faiths. By
Christian mystics, the compassion energy that stems from *bodhi* is
taken to be God's love; Sufis and Hindus have somewhat similar
conceptions of it. By Buddhists it is known as *mahā karunā* (great
compassion) and, in its primary form, is held to be the dynamic
principle of *bodhi* and therefore essential for demolishing the illusory
barriers between minds and that One Mind of which the universe's
transient forms are creations. Whether or not the nature and functioning of *karunā* are properly understood, its beneficent activity is a
matter of direct experience not disputed by those who have attained to
a large measure of intuitive wisdom.

(ii) One must also be able to accept – though without troubling
much about explanations, which in any case are apt to vary – the
effectiveness of the Mahayana practice of embodying *mahā karunā* for
yogic purposes in one or more of the traditional semi-
anthropomorphic forms well suited to our human habits of conceptualisation – it being understood that the forms themselves are mental
constructs and that if, say, horses are able to envisage some sort of
parallel notion, *mahā karunā* is probably embodied by them in the
form of a horse (such a form being indeed one of those traditionally
attributed to Kuan Yin Bodhisattva). The extent to which such

embodiments are beings existing independently or not independently of the minds of the individuals who invoke them is a matter of speculation with no direct bearing upon effective practice of the yoga.

(iii) One who undertakes this type of yoga, whether for his own benefit or on behalf of others, must himself be a compassionate person or, at the very least, undertake henceforth to assist sentient beings as far as lies within his power and to refrain scrupulously from deliberately harming them even in thought, let alone by his actions.

(b) SOME TRADITIONAL EMBODIMENTS OF MAHĀ KARUNĀ

This energy in its primary form is embodied in the Celestial Buddha Amitābha (Tibetan, Opagme; Chinese Ô-mi-to Fu). Yogic practice centred on this embodiment is directed at rebirth in a Pure Land (often equated with pure Mind free from all impediments arising from ego-delusion). In its secondary form, it is embodied in the Celestial Bodhisattva Avalokiteśvara, also known as Avalokita (Tibetan, Chenresigs; Chinese, Kuan Yin or Kuan Shih Yin), who is credited with a Pure Land function identical with that of Amitābha Buddha, but also with that of curing or ameliorating worldly troubles experienced in the present life.

In its tertiary form, *mahā karunā* is embodied in Tara (Tibetan, Tara or Dolma; Chinese, Lü Tu Mu), who chiefly performs the second of those functions. Each of the three forms is envisaged as being intimately connected with the others, Avalokita as emanating from Amitābha, Tara as emanating from Avalokita. Each fulfils certain yogic and psychological needs.

In what follows, we shall be concerned with the secondary embodiment, Avalokita/Kuan Yin, and solely with the function of curing or ameliorating worldly troubles, this being a matter about which I feel somewhat better qualified to write. During the greater part of my life, I have employed the invocation to and mantra of Avalokita/Kuan Yin for a variety of purposes. For purely personal reasons, I have added to these the mantra and yogic evocation of Tara as aids to my own safety, well-being and yogic progress, having been given by my lama this beautiful, fun-loving, infinitely compassionate being as my main *yidam* (indwelling deity or 'Buddha-in-my heart') and have thenceforth invoked Avalokita/Kuan Yin mainly on behalf of others. However, yogically, there is no fundamental difference between these forms and it would be an unnecessary complication to introduce the separate practices relating to each of them here. Avalokita/Kuan Yin can be invoked very effectively both on behalf of others and on one's own.

Avalokita Bodhisattva is chiefly depicted and visualised in three of his innumerable forms, of which the first and second are common among Tibetan Buddhists; the first and third, among Chinese, Japanese, Korean and Vietnamese Buddhists. They are:

(i) A standing figure with eleven heads, a thousand eyes and a thousand arms, symbolising simultaneous perception of the sorrows of all sentient beings and infinite power to cure, ameliorate and comfort. This symbolism brings to mind the meaning of Avalokita/ Kuan Yin's name – Hearer of the Cries of the World. This form is normally visualised during recitation of the Dhāraṇī (or Mantra) of Great Compassion and also of the Heart Sutra as well as during yogic practices performed on behalf of the welfare and happiness of all sentient beings.

(ii) A figure seated in the lotus posture with one head and four arms, two extended in the mudrā of blessing, two held in front of the breast with the hands cupping the 'wish-fulfilling gem', symbol of liberation attained through the union of wisdom and compassion. It is the form appropriate to recitation of the mantra *OṀ MAṆI PADMÉ HŪṀ*.

(iii) A standing or seated figure in the form of a lovely lady, generally robed and hooded in white (or blue), lips curved in a tender smile, eyes filled with pity or half closed in the bliss of meditation. This form, virtually unknown in Tibet, probably combines Avalokita/Kuan Yin and Tara into one figure and is the principal form of the Bodhisattva envisaged in countries lying further to the east, notably China and Japan.

For the purpose of the following yogas, any of these forms will be equally effective, unless a specific form is indicated in my text; but people working as a group should, of course, envisage the same form simultaneously – this can be decided upon in advance. The forms, after all, are mental constructs, whereas the reality is abstract, formless, a marvellous activity latent in Mind. The power of *mahā karunā* is infinite, the visualised embodiments belong to the category of *upaya* (skilful means). Whichever embodiment is invoked, response is certain, if the longing for *mahā karunā* is heartfelt and the individuals who evoke it endeavour at all times to exercise compassion towards all sentient beings. The degree of effectiveness steadily increases with long and frequent practice over months and years. As the results become more striking, the adept should guard against drawing unnecessary attention to his success, much less boast of it, for he is no more than an imperfect vehicle through which the *mahā karunā* embodied in Avalokita/Kuan Yin operates. Any attempt to employ this power for self-aggrandisement will surely result in its diminution. Latent in Mind and therefore in our minds, it lies always at hand for those prepared to use it beneficially without unnecessary display.

(c) TECHNIQUES OF COMPASSION YOGA AND SOME APPLICATIONS

From the first, the adept should be constantly alert to the sufferings around him. Invariably, when he chances to see a person or animal in distress, he should utter softly and unostentatiously the invocation 'Homage to the Greatly Compassionate Avalokiteśvara Bodhisattva' (or 'Na-mo Ta-pei Kuan-Shih-Yin P'u-sa'), or else the mantra *OṀ MANI PADMĖ HŪṀ*, accompanying this by a brief visualisation of the Bodhisattva coupled with a profound aspiration for the well-being of the sufferer. One consequence of doing so will be that the adept's alertness to the sufferings around him will be a perpetual stimulus to the generation of *bodhi-citta* (compassionate heart/mind), which is essential to Enlightenment. A more immediate consequence will be that the power of the invocation or mantra – a power that increases with frequency of utterance over the years – will bring about actual amelioration of the sufferer's condition, varying from a passing sensation of comfort and well-being to diminution or disappearance of the cause of suffering, depending on the heaviness of the sufferer's own *karma*. Examples of sufferings which in the past we may barely have allowed to impinge upon our consciousness include a blind or crippled person encountered in the street, a mangy dog, a traveller held up by a stalled engine, the victim of a motor accident on the far side of the road, an unhappy or frightened child, a baby screaming in the night to whom no one seems to pay attention, a bird with a broken wing, a person cruelly snubbed or scolded. It is not often possible by yogic means to counteract another's *karma* to the extent of causing the blind to see or the lame to run; yet it is astonishing how often perceptible results supervene immediately, for example the frightened child, unaware of what has been done for him, smiles, the baby's screams very rapidly subside.

With practice, the invocation or the mantra comes immediately to the adept's lips in times of crisis, whether he is awake or sleeping. By its means, his car, having swerved and hurtled towards a roadside ditch to avoid a speeding lorry, is brought under control just in the nick of time to prevent grave harm to the occupants; or a fearsome nightmare abruptly changes course and the terror promptly subsides. (In another book, I have described how the hellish 'trip' brought on by my one experience with a psychedelic drug was transformed in a flash, by a single utterance of my *yidam*'s mantra, into a joyous and wisdom-fraught experience.) People long familiar with the practice are able to recount literally hundreds of examples of physical and psychic dangers overcome by evoking the power of *mahā karunā*.

The same technique can be used most effectively for comforting frightened or grief-stricken people and animals whom one knows well enough to take in one's arms or establish some other physical contact. In this case, one repeats the invocation or the mantra for as long as possible in a soothing voice, meanwhile visualising the Bodhisattva in the form of a lovely lady holding in her right hand a vase containing the 'sweet dew' of wisdom-compassion, a few drops of which are seen to fall upon the sufferer's head. If the sufferer, once he has recovered his wits, can be induced to join in the invocation, so much the better. An aged Mongolian lama enabled me to recover within a few hours from a malady that had caused me to lose consciousness and fall from my mule while on a long journey, simply by sitting by my bed and soothingly muttering the mantra OM MANI PADME HŪM until I fell asleep.

A more elaborate technique, combining utterance of the invocation or of the mantra with a detailed visualisation of the Bodhisattva, can be used for curing anxiety, hysteria, and even grave physical or mental illness in oneself or others. Various ways of using it are set forth in section II, B, 6.

(d) A YOGIC RITE

One who desires to attain full proficiency as a vehicle of the Bodhisattva's compassion should perform the following rite not less than once a day, abbreviating it only if strictly necessary. It has been adapted from various more complicated rites set forth in the Chinese monastic rubric and combined with an all-important visualisation practice that probably derives from the teachings of the Mi Tsung, or Esoteric Sect, during the time of its ascendancy more than a thousand years ago. Though tantric in character, the visualisation practice has been handed down through non-initiates and is therefore open to everybody. The whole rite can be performed by an individual or a group, the pronoun 'I' or 'we' being used throughout as appropriate.

(i) Facing a likeness of the Buddha and/or of Avalokita/Kuan Yin Bodhisattva, bow low and plant three, five, seven or nine incense sticks upright in an ash-packed incense-burner, ceremoniously using both hands to insert them one by one. (This can be done by the group leader with the others watching.) The action is accompanied by the following recitation:

> *We prostrate ourselves*
> *And offer incense*
> *As a dharma-offering.*
> *May these clouds of perfumed smoke*
> *Interfuse the universe*
> *And every Buddha-land*
> *In the form of countless*
> *Precious offerings!*

(followed by three prostrations).

(ii) The act of taking refuge in the Enlightened One, the Sacred Teaching and the Sacred Community is performed by chanting:

> *We go for refuge to the Buddha*

(one prostration)

> *We go for refuge to the Dharma*

(one prostration)

> *We go for refuge to the Sangha*

(one prostration)

(iii) Standing and visualising the Bodhisattva in thousand-eyed, thousand-armed form, recite the invocation:

> *Homage to the Greatly Compassionate Kuan Yin Bodhisattva*

or

> *Na-mo Ta-pei Kuan-Shih-Yin P'u-sa*

(three, seven, twenty-one or one hundred and eight times, followed by three prostrations).

(iv) Seated in meditation posture and visualising the Bodhisattva as before, recite:

It is written that the Bodhisattva, in the presence of the Buddha, enunciated these vows:
'World Honoured, should any being recite and cleave to the sacred Dhāranī of Great Compassion and yet fall into one of the three evil states of existence, I vow not to enter upon Supreme Enlightenment.

'Should any being recite and cleave to the sacred Dhāranī of Great Compassion and yet not be born in any Buddhaland, I vow not to enter upon Supreme Enlightenment.

'Should any being recite and cleave to the sacred Dhāranī of Great Compassion and yet not achieve the eloquence (born of) limitless samadhi, I vow not to enter upon Supreme Enlightenement.

'Should any being recite and cleave to the sacred Dhāranī of Great Compassion and yet not obtain in this very life the fruits of all he desires, then he cannot have been (properly reciting and cleaving to) the Dhāranī of the Heart of Great Compassion. He should put away wrong-doing and put away insincerity.'

Now recite the *dhāranī* (using the following Sanskrit text, or the Chinese or Japanese text, both of which are to be found in romanised form in the appendix):

'Namo ratna-trayāya namah ārya avalokiteśvarāya bodhisattvāya mahasattvāya mahākarunikāya oṃ sabalavati śudhanatasya namaskrivanimaṃ ārya avalokiteśvara lamtabha namo nīlakantha śrīmahapataśami sarvatodhuśupheṃ aśiyum sarvasada nama bhaga mabhatetu tadyathā oṃ āvaloki lokate kalati eśili mahābodhisattva sabho sabho mara mara maśi ridhayuṃ guru guru gamam turu turu bhaśiyati mahā bhaśiyati dhara dhara dhirini śvaraya jala jala mama bhamara mudhili edhyehi śina śina alaśim bhalaśari bhaśa bhaśim bharaśaya hulu hulu pra hulu hulu śrī sara sara siri siri suru suru budhi budhi budhaya budhaya maitriye nīlakantha triśarana bhayamaṇa svāhā sitaya svāhā mahā sitaya svāhā sitayaye śvaraya svāhā nīlakaṇṭhi svāhā pranila svāhā śrī sidha mukhaya svāhā sarva mahā astaya svāhā cakra astaya svāhā padma keśaya svāhā nīlakaṇṭhe paṇṭalaya svāhā mobholiśaṅkaraye svāhā namo ratna-trayāya namah ārya avalokita īśvaraya svāhā oṃ sidhyantu mantra pataye svāhā'

(three, seven, twenty-one, one hundred and eight or 1,080 times, according to circumstances).

Recite:

When Avalokita Bodhisattva had finished uttering this dhāranī for the first time in the presence of the Buddha, the great earth underwent six convulsions; jewelled flowers rained down from the sky; the Buddhas of the ten quarters of the universe rejoiced, and evil beings shuddered.

Silently reflect that the fruits of uttering and cleaving to this *dhāranī* include a heart/mind characterised by vast compassion, equanimity, freedom from defilements and attachments, ability to contemplate the void, reverence, humility, no confusion, no disposition to cling to dualistic views, and a plenitude of unexcelled *bodhi*; as well as avoidance of all forms of untimely death, and attainment of rebirth under conditions highly conducive to wise and virtuous living and leading to Enlightenment. However, to achieve all these in full, one must first have taken the Bodhisattva Vow to deliver all sentient beings, and one must at all times observe the precepts against killing, stealing, improper sex, lying and intoxication.

Silently repeat these words:

I and all sentient beings from beginningless time have been involved in the creation of many kinds of evil karma-forming activity obstructive of Enlightenment. Ignorant of the Buddhas and of the Way to liberation, we have wandered through repeated births and deaths without knowledge of the marvellous principles enunciated by Shakyamuni Buddha. Now in the presence of the Bodhisattva of Compassion and the Buddhas of the ten quarters of the universe, I [or we] express remorse on behalf of all living beings for these failings, desiring only to assist them in overcoming hindrances to Enlightenment.

(v) Still seated, recite the Heart Sutra *three times*, slowly and with clear insight into its teaching, which is of a highly esoteric character. All the ordinary teachings of the Buddha are here transcended in the light of intuition of the void nature of existence. The five *skandhas* or components of an individual's seeming personality are proclaimed to be void, as are the six sense organs (including mind), the six forms of sense perception and the six types of consciousness to which they give rise. Even such fundamental teachings are negated as the twelvefold chain of causation leading from primordial ignorance, through becoming, etc., to decay, death and rebirth; the four Noble Truths (that existence is inseparable from suffering/frustration, that the cause of suffering/frustration is inordinate desire, that the remedy is cessation of inordinate desire/aversion, and that this results from treading the Noble Eightfold Path requiring right attitudes and conduct of both body and mind); and the attainment of Nirvana through the exercise of wisdom. All these teachings, though absolutely valid at the level of relative truth apparent to us all, are found to have no pertinence once the void nature of reality has been fully realised and conceptualisation transcended. The reference at the end of the sutra to uttering the Mantra of Highest Wisdom means not that one just utters it, but that he *lives* the mantra by perceiving the voidness of all concepts, entities and beings without exception. The exoteric teachings of the Buddha must most certainly not be abandoned until the intuitive experience of voidness leads to brilliant, unwavering perception of the pure, boundless, shining void. The words to be recited are as follows:

Homage to the Sutra of the Heart of Highest Wisdom!

Avalokiteśvara Bodhisattva, while engaged in deep practice of the highest wisdom, perceived that all the five aggregates are void, and thereby passed beyond all forms of suffering. O Sariputra, form differs not from void, nor void from form. Form IS void; void IS form. With feelings, perceptions, conditionings and consciousness it is the same. Sariputra, all these are marked by emptiness, neither coming into being nor ceasing to be, neither foul nor pure, neither increasing nor diminishing. Therefore within the void there are no form, no feelings, perceptions, conditionings or consciousness; no eyes, ears, nose, tongue, body or mind; no form, sound, smell, taste, touch or thought; nor any of the others from eye-consciousness to mind-consciousness. There is neither ignorance nor extinction of ignorance, nor any of the other [twelve links of causation] down to decay and death. There is no suffering, no cause, no remedy, no path [thereto]. There is no wisdom, no attainment. Because there is nothing to be attained, Bodhisattvas relying on this highest wisdom are free from hindrances of mind. Being rid of these hindrances, they have no fear, are free from all upsets and delusions, and in the end attain Nirvana. It is by relying on this highest wisdom that all Buddhas of the past, the present and the future achieve Supreme Enlightenment. Therefore do we know that the highest wisdom is a great and sacred mantra, a great mantra of knowledge, a mantra unsurpassed, unequalled. It can terminate all suffering truly and unfailingly. Therefore utter this Mantra of Highest Wisdom thus — 'Gaté, gaté, pāragaté, pārasamgaté, bodhi, svāhā!' [Gone, gone, gone beyond, wholly gone beyond! Enlightenment! Svāhā!]

Homage to the Sutra of the Heart of Highest Wisdom.
(Versions of this sutra, romanised for recitation in Chinese and
Japanese instead of English will be found in the appendix.)

(vi) Still seated, allow the visualisation of the Bodhisattva in
thousand-eyed, thousand-armed form to fade from consciousness
preparatory to the following visualisation. What comes next is the
most vital part of the yogic rite.

Try to visualise pure void – nothing, emptiness. Presently this
emptiness is replaced by a vista of calm ocean lit by a full moon close to
the horizon. The sea is silver with little white-topped waves, the sky
blue-black, the white moon bright but not dazzling. You stare at the
moon a long time, feeling increasingly calm and happy. Then the
moon beings to diminish in size, growing ever brighter, until it
resembles a pearl so bright that one can only just bear to look at it.
After a while, the pearl expands until it is no longer a pearl but a
radiant nimbus, in the heart of which stands a lovely lady robed and
hooded in gleaming white, her feet resting on a lotus that floats upon
the waves. Every detail of her form is clearly seen, for her face and
form are illumined respectively by a glowing white halo and nimbus;
even her garments emit light. You are no longer conscious of a great
stretch of sea between you and the Bodhisattva Kuan Yin. Mysteriously she has advanced to within a few feet of where you are sitting.
Her lovely smile and whole expression reveal the joy she feels in the
company of those who have evoked her in order to draw upon the
power of compassion. If you keep very calm, just whispering her
name over and over, and making no attempt to constrain her to stay,
she may of her own accord remain for what will seem a long, long
time. Presently, however, her whole form will diminish to the size of a
mote of dust, and then vanish together with sky and sea. All that
remains then is lovely, shining space extending in all directions
without end. This vision of space will stay long if, by then, you have
become so forgetful of yourself as to be united with it in subject-
objectless unity. At this point, there should be no thought of you and
space – just space, no you.

(vii) Conclusion of the rite. Standing, recite the formula:

Homage to the Greatly Compassionate Kuan Yin Bodhisattva

or

Na-mo Ta-pei Kuan-Shih-Yin P'u-sa

(three times, each accompanied by one prostration)

We go for refuge to the Buddha

(one prostration)

We go for refuge to the Dharma

(one prostration)

We go for refuge to the Sangha

(one prostration)

(End of the rite)

A simplified variant of this rite is to substitute continuous chanting of the formula contained in (iii) for all the parts from (iv) to (vi). If this is done rhythmically, it may lead to an expanded state of consciousness; but it is generally held that frequent repetition of the Dhāranī of Great Compassion is a more powerful and effective means of developing *mahā karunā* and overcoming obstacles than simple invocation.

Another and altogether excellent variant is to substitute for triple recitation of (v) the Heart Sutra a single or triple recitation of the poem from the Lotus Sutra that forms Appendix III. This is particularly appropriate when the whole rite is being performed to ward off danger or disaster.

(e) A STORY

Stories of miraculous response to recitation of the Dhāranī of Great Compassion are common throughout the countries of East Asia. The following is a typical example. In 1933, when fierce hostilities broke out between China and Japan in the neighbourhood of Shanghai, several of the city's suburbs were flattened by intensive bombing followed by raging fires. Unaware that things were about to come to such a pass, four middle-aged ladies gathered one afternoon in the upper storey of a small two-storeyed house there intending to play mah-jong far into the night. They were worldly-minded ladies without much thought for anything besides their own pleasure; when bombs started falling around them and flames shot up from neighbouring buildings, they were beside themselves with terror, for there seemed to be no way of escaping a fiery death. The only other person present in the house was an elderly *amah* (maid), whom the owner of the place was fond of describing to her cronies as 'no better than a half-wit'. When the first bombs crashed down, this thin, shabby, grey-haired old creature came running in to be at hand should her mistress need her, but did not join the ladies in their lamentations. If the others had paid any attention to her, they might have been put to shame by her unruffled calm.

'Old Father Heaven!' shrieked the most elegant of the guests, forgetting the dignified reserve on which she had hitherto prided herself. 'This is what comes of living frivolously without respect for the gods or the least effort to placate malevolent demons. Now we shall be roasted alive, and who knows how long it will take to die?'

'*Aiyah*!' cried another. 'Don't say it! My brains have begun to fry already. My skull seems . . .'

'Enough!' moaned a third. 'Have you no pity? Look at our poor hostess! You have driven her two souls from her body with your irresponsible talk.'

This seemed not unlikely, for the corpulent Mrs Ch'ên had slumped forward, face white as a ghost's, and brought her chin so sharply in contact with the marble table-top as to send some of the mah-jong tiles tumbling to the floor. A stream of blood issuing from her lips made it fairly certain she had bitten her tongue at the moment of fainting away. As for the others, their agonised twitter, punctuated by the crash of masonry as house after house disintegrated around them, continued unabated for a while. Then one by one they fell silent and sat staring in amazement at the 'dim-witted' countrywoman they had been in the habit of treating with careless contempt. Unnoticed until then, she had fallen to her knees; her expression was placid and a smile hovered on her lips as, in surprisingly vigorous tones, of which they had not deemed such a self-effacing creature capable, she intoned very slowly the words of the ancient Dhāranī of Great Compassion – '. . . *SŪ FŬ LÀ YÄ, DSŌ LÀ DSŌ LÀ, MŌ MŌ FÀ MŌ LÄ . . .*'.

Only one of the ladies present had as much as a vague idea as to what these strange un-Chinese sounding syllables might portend; priding themselves on being thoroughly up to date, they had not – unless in early childhood – heard anything of the kind, or, if they had heard monks reciting mantras at funeral ceremonies, they had not paid the least attention. Now, however, immensely impressed by they knew not what, they began chorusing the unfamiliar syllables in the pauses which the illiterate *amah* considerately prolonged so as to encourage the others to join in. In a little while, even Mrs Ch'ên had recovered sufficiently to add her quota in a quavering voice. Unnoticed by them, the bombing had ceased, but the crackle of flames, the rumble of falling buildings, the screams of the injured and dying rose from very close by, and from time to time dense black smoke came driving in through the windows from which all the glass had long ago fallen away. Curiously, an extraordinary stillness had settled upon the room. Anyone entering just then would have found the women uttering the resonant syllables in voices so calm that they might have been tellers totting up figures in a bank. Over and over again the mantra was repeated by five people totally oblivious of the lurid flames without and the stench of roasting flesh that mingled with the other odours of dire destruction. Gradually these various horrors abated, but the voices continued zealously – '. . . *POO YĂ MŌ NŌ, SŌ PŎ HŌ, SHĬ TŌ YĂ . . .*'.

After several hours, they one by one fell silent from sheer exhaustion, yet looking more at peace with themselves than on any previous occasion. Now they noticed that the sun had risen upon the scene of devastation around them. Bowing even lower to the old *amah* than to their hostess, Mrs Ch'ên, the three ladies who lived elsewhere sallied forth amidst the smoking ruins, praying that their own quarter of the city was still standing. To left, to right, in front, behind stretched unending scenes of desolation; scarcely a building stood and none of these few was by any means virtually undamaged, with the exception of the house where they had passed that fearful night protected by the faith of a 'half-wit' in the saving power of the Compassionate Bodhisattva, Kuan Yin!

The point of this story is *not* that the Dhāraṇi of Great Compassion is a magic spell able to protect whoever recites it in the midst of dire peril, though indeed it may sometimes appear to act like that, if one or more of those who utter it possesses, perhaps unknown to himself, what are called 'good roots'. It is probable that the allegedly half-witted servant was a simple person with great integrity of character who had mastered the mantra by frequent repetition accompanied by strict adherence to the precepts and a genuine desire to be of service to all sentient beings. In that case, the compassionate heart of the humble (and, it may be, far from bright) old woman naturally constituted an admirable vehicle through which *mahā karunā* could flow unimpeded by obstacles of any kind.

6

Cleansing and Healing Yoga

(a) INTRODUCTORY

Proper understanding of the techniques described in this section
requires familiarity with the ideas set forth in sections II, B, 5, (a), (b)
and (c) above.

(b) SELF-CLEANSING

The state of mind attainable by this practice transcends that of a
Christian spiritually cleansed in the confessional, or of a patient
returned to mental wholeness on his analyst's couch; it dispels every
kind of psychical burden without resource to priest, doctor or external deity. I have based this simplified form of a traditional technique
partly on the superbly effective method of self-cleansing (by means of
the Vajrasattva rite) employed by Tibetan lamas, and partly on a
Chinese-type visualisation of the Bodhisattva Kuan Yin. As the
former would require initiation prior to instruction, I have had to
devise an analogous method suitable for those not immediately in a
position to obtain initiation. Such a welding of elements derived
severally from Tibetan and Chinese sources fully accords with Chinese tradition; for, since the vanishing from China a thousand years ago
of the Mi Tsung or Esoteric Sect of Buddhism, individual Chinese
teachers have frequently borrowed from Tibetan and Mongolian
lamas to compensate for the gap left by the disruption of the Mi Tsung
lineage. The Chinese commonly invoke Kuan Yin, Bodhisattva of
Compassion, to ameliorate or cure distress of *every* kind whatsoever;
moreover, the core of the present rite – visualisation of the
Bodhisattva emerging from a moon shining down upon a limitless
ocean – is undoubtedly a survival from Chinese Mi Tsung practice.

No innovations are involved in the present use of it, beyond applying that visualisation *specifically to self-cleansing* in a manner reminiscent of the Tibetan Vajrasattva rite. My venturing to make even such a limited use in this context of a tantric technique intended for initiates is, I believe, permissible, as my teacher, Dodrup Chen Rinpoche, graciously authorised me to rely upon my own discretion as to how much to say or leave unsaid in my writings on tantric subjects, and I have scrupulously avoided including anything analogous to the more secret aspects of the Vajrasattva cleansing practice.

Preferably at *regular* and not infrequent intervals (three months at the very most), everyone who practises yogic meditation should set aside a session for self-cleansing. The adept, having lighted incense, prostrated himself thrice in homage to the Triple Gem[1] and taken up his usual meditation posture, reflects: 'Here am I, feet firmly set upon the Way but beset by formidable shortcomings arising from my load of *karma*. During the past week' – month, two or three months, as the case may be – 'I have often allowed my thoughts to wander during my yogic meditations or performed them perfunctorily. Many, many times by day or night, when not engaged in meditating, I have relaxed awareness and allowed myself to behave in ways' – these may be dwelt upon specifically – 'ill-befitting a follower of the Way. For all my unskilful, *karma*-forming actions of body, speech and mind I am truly sorry. I long to be rid of their fruits, the better to reach Enlightenment and thus become an undiminishing source of the wisdom and compassion so direly needed by myriads of beings now revolving helplessly in the round of birth and death.' (Note that remorse should not stem from egoistic concern over one's own situation and its pains, but wholly from eagerness to be of unlimited help to others.)

Having sorrowfully reflected on these matters and fully determined to do better from now on, the adept invokes Kuan Yin by reciting over and over again the formula: 'Homage to the Greatly Compassionate Kuan Yin Bodhisattva' or 'Na-mo Ta-pei Kuan-Shih-Yin P'u-sa'. Uttering the invocation slowly and solemnly, he presently visualises a calm ocean spreading to the horizon in all directions, in the midst of which he finds himself seated as though floating weightlessly upon the water.

A full moon, risen only recently and still not far above the ocean's rim, softly illuminates the scene. Before long, Kuan Yin Bodhisattva appears within it in the form of a beautiful lady clad in white robes (see

[1]The prostrations may be followed, if desired, by employing the offering mudrās described in section II, B, 3, (c).

illustration), whereat the moon disc is transformed into a nimbus of white light radiating from her body which, like her robes, possesses its own effulgence. Her feet rest upon a giant white lotus, its petals tinged with pinkish red. After a while, this lotus skims smoothly across the intervening waves until the Bodhisattva stands only a few feet in front of the adept, gazing down at him with a joyful smile. Next, a long-continuing stream of dazzling white light issues from her forehead and, entering through the crown of his head, begins to push its way slowly downwards, driving before it all the evils afflicting his mind and body – innumerable shortcomings that lead to *karma*-forming action and thus to endless wandering through the round of birth and death, as well as pains, sorrows, anxieties, fierce passions, ignorance, stupidity and every kind of malady both mental and physical. These he now visualises as a noxious stream of heavy black liquid flowing down to and out through the lower part of his body, sinking into the ocean beneath him, and being greedily gobbled up by a host of demons in the shape of vile sea-monsters who have rushed from all directions to take part in this horrid feast. (This part of the visualisation should on no account be omitted, lest the evils expelled contaminate the surroundings and do harm to whatever small creatures may be there.)

The white radiance having gradually reached down to the tips of the adept's fingers and toes, filling every nook and cranny of his being without exception, he comes to resemble a crystal vessel brimming with glowing effulgence. Thus he remains for a while, rejoicing in the compassion so freely and joyfully vouchsafed and continuing without pause to utter the invocation, which should not cease until the very end of the rite. (Alternatively he may, if he wishes, begin by reciting the invocation three, nine or twenty-one times and then substitute utterance of the mantra *OM MANI PADMÉ HŪM*, returning to the invocation only at the end when he rises to prostrate himself.)

When quiet, joyous contemplation of the Bodhisattva has been maintained for as long as possible, the adept visualises her body as gradually becoming fainter, until at last it is indistinguishable from the moon-like nimbus which, contracting to a point of white fire no larger than a pin-head, presently vanishes. Even after this, he remains seated for a while, revelling in a sensation of weightlessness and freedom so powerful that he may feel he must exercise a little restraint to prevent himself from levitating or flying off into the air. Should the impulse to levitate be strong, he should resist it, as it would not do at this stage to give way to such a feeling.

To close the rite, he emerges from his visualisation, rises to his feet

and performs three prostrations accompanied by the invocation to
Kuan Yin and by heartfelt aspirations for the happiness and welfare of
all beings. Finally, he makes three further prostrations in homage to
the Triple Gem.

(c) SELF-HEALING

This practice should be undertaken with caution, that is to say after
careful consideration as to the nature of the complaint to be healed. If
the malady is a long-standing one, self-healing through the power of
the Compassionate Bodhisattva should not be attempted for a reason
that will soon become clear.

When, during the second of my visits to the Himalayan region, I
was introduced at the little hillside town of Kalimpong to Dudjom
Rinpoche, whose pupil I was soon to become, I was surprised to learn
that this great master of yogic practice had been suffering for many
decades from an intermittently acute form of asthma. Surely, I
reflected, so notable a yogin has means to rid himself of a tiresome
complaint that often interferes with his plans for doing various kinds
of important work? This was not a matter I felt able to put to him with
propriety, as he did not then know me well and might suppose me
capable of the insolence of calling into question the extent of his yogic
powers. Instead, I sought an answer in what I had already learnt of
Buddhism during my years in China. There, on the one hand, I had
heard stories of wellnigh miraculous cures and even witnessed a few
with my own eyes; but, on the other, I had noticed that famous
Dharma Masters do get ill just like other people, though somewhat
more rarely due to their abstaining from all kinds of emotional and
bodily excess, and to the healthy mode of living pursued in mountain
monasteries and retreats. While living for some months in the Hua
T'ing Monastery near Kunming, I had been distressed to discover
that many of the monks there had large open sores on their bodies.
Having at that time less faith in Chinese medicine that I developed
later, I took one of them down into the city to be examined by a
refugee physician from Vienna. After a cursory examination, the
doctor made a gesture of helplessness and explained that there was
nothing he could do, as the monk was clearly a victim of under-
nourishment – the result of the impoverished state of Hua T'ing
Monastery during the Second World War, when the whole country
was suffering from the effects of the Japanese occupation of its most
fruitful regions.

Thinking over these matters, I came to the conclusion that physical maladies can be divided, from a Buddhist point of view, into two categories – those forming part of the karmic load resulting from unskilful actions of body, speech and mind performed in this and previous lives; and those due to concurrent causes. I realised that so great a yogin as Dudjom Rinpoche could probably use his undoubted powers to cure his malady, but that he might not wish to do so as, if it were due to *karma* accumulated in a previous life, its cure would result in the *karma*'s working itself out in some other unpleasant way. Karmic accumulations cannot be effaced either by virtuous living or by an act of will, but have to be worked out. The correct yogic means of overcoming them is to refrain from actions that will add to the load and thus prevent its gradual diminution. On the other hand, illnesses due to concurrent causes not directly related to the operation of heavy *karma* stemming from a previous life do lend themselves to treatment by yogic means, which I believe would have been suitable for the malady afflicting many of the monks in Hua T'ing Monastery.

To assess the category to which a particular illness belongs is no easy matter. As a rough guide, I would suggest that long-standing or frequently recurrent maladies be looked upon as due to karmic causes, whereas those due to present or recent circumstances be regarded as suitable for cure by yogic means. In particular, illnesses caused by unhealthy states of mind, by tension, nervousness, anxiety, depression, fear, intemperance (for example with regard to anger, sex, drugs or liquor), are highly susceptible to cure by yogic means. To avoid disappointment, one must enter upon the practice in the knowledge that some ills are incurable by this means, or rather that their cure would not result in overall good for the patient. Nevertheless, once an attempt to cure has been decided upon, it should be entered into in a thoroughly optimistic state of mind. Cures by yogic means cannot be wrought in a state of doubt.

What may loosely be termed 'self-healing', though in fact it is healing through the power of *karunā* embodied in the form of Kuan Yin Bodhisattva, requires performance of a rite exactly like that for self-cleansing as set forth in section (b) above, except for four important differences: (i) It should be performed not at regular intervals spaced out over a long period, but intensively – say, once, twice or thrice a day until the malady subsides or becomes greatly ameliorated. (ii) The reflection on past shortcomings and forming of a determination to do better in future should be replaced by reflection on the sufferings of all sentient beings, during which individual examples of human and animal suffering are brought vividly to mind, and followed by heartfelt aspiration for the welfare and happiness of those particular individuals and all other beings. (iii) During the visualisation of Kuan Yin Bodhisattva, the consciousness is directed to the seat of the particular malady to be expelled. Should it happen to be a localised malady, the mind should be fixed upon its removal by the influx of white radiance to the part of the body afflicted, which drives it down to the lower orifices in the form of evil liquid and expels it into the mouths of the sea-monsters. (A psychological ill may be visualised as residing in the head. If the seat of the ill is in an arm or a leg, a small technical difficulty will be experienced, but can be resolved in one of two ways. Either the dark liquid can be visualised as being forced out by the white radiance through the fingers or toes instead of through the lower orifices of the body; or else the radiance can be visualised as forcing its way *past* the afflicted spot, reaching the fingers or toes and then *returning* to drive the malady by a convenient route down to the lower orifices.) (iv) The aspirations for the happiness and welfare of all beings that accompany the prostrations at the end should be replaced by aspirations mentally worded or actually voiced somewhat on the following lines: 'May all sentient beings afflicted by ills of mind or body be freed from those afflictions and attain to radiant health!'

(d) HEALING OTHERS (INCLUDING GROUP HEALING)

To a considerable extent, the same limitation on the kinds of malady suitable for yogic treatment applies here as that discussed in the section on self-healing; yet, in this case, the limitation is possibly less absolute. If a completely disinterested person (one free from desire for recompense or for fame as a healer) evokes the power of *karunā* on behalf of another being, the merit of his generous aspiration may be expected to have at least some effect in counterbalancing the patient's evil *karma*, particularly if his own stock of merit (a term for accumulations of '*good karma*') is large and he is only too happy to transfer some of it for the purpose of effecting a cure. Also, one may suppose that the power of *karunā* embodied in Kuan Yin Bodhisattva will respond very actively to a truly compassionate intention, so that even a person of rather small merit may succeed in evoking that power on behalf of another. To accomplish a transfer of merit, all that is needed is a simple act of will by the one who has accumulated it; indeed, there are Buddhists who perform such an act daily as part of their regular devotions in some such words as 'I beg to offer the merit of all good acts of body, speech and mind for the benefit of sentient beings everywhere.' To make a transfer of merit specific, one should reflect:'I offer merit for the benefit of so-and-so. May he be healed of his malady.' There is nothing miraculous about such transfers; our minds being indivisible from Mind are, except at the level of relative truth where dualistic distinctions hold good, indivisible from one another; hence sincere aspirations on the part of one person naturally affect others (as, alas, do evil thoughts as well). Such interchanges happen continually, which accounts for the atmosphere of good or evil one senses upon certain occasions in gatherings of people. Furthermore, as I discovered during some of my seminars in North America, if a group of people simultaneously evoke the power of *karunā* embodied in Kuan Yin Bodhisattva on behalf of someone sick or injured, their combined endeavour is more effective than that of a single person.

For an individual who seeks to heal another by evoking the power of *karunā*, the method is similar to that for self-healing, except that the preliminary aspiration, the actual visualisation rite and the concluding aspiration should all be directed solely towards the person to be healed. Thus, during the visualisation, the stream of white radiance issuing from the Bodhisattva's forehead enters not the body of the meditator (who need not be present in the picture), but that of the patient, who should be present if possible, and in any case visualised as sitting or reclining upon the surface of the ocean in front of the Bodhisattva. The stream of light is seen to enter through the crown of his head and gradually pervade his whole body, from which his malady is expelled in the form of an evil black liquid that is swallowed by the sea-monsters. Moreover, if the patient is to be present in person or can be notified in advance of the exact time of the healing rite, he should, if his condition has left him mentally alert and not too weak, be taught the healing method and himself take part in the invocation of Kuan Yin and subsequent visualisation. In such a case, he naturally visualises the stream of radiance entering his own body. The patient's co-operation in the healing will greatly add to the degree of success, but he should not be urged to co-operate unless this is warranted by his physical and mental condition at the time. Should he wish to co-operate, but not be in a fit state to perform the full visualisation, a middle course is for him to recite the invocation to Kuan Yin or the mantra *OṀ MANI PADMÉ HŪṀ* with his thoughts quietly concentrated upon her form.

For group healing by this means, the patient should, if possible, be seated or recline in the centre of a circle formed by the group. Whether or not he is actually present, the members of the group should visualise him seated alone upon the water facing the Bodhisattva. Though this mental picture occurs simultaneously in their minds and they are thus creating it, they do not need to visualise themselves as being part of the scene – all they see is the limitless ocean, the moon, the Bodhisattva and the patient. A method of synchronising such a group activity is given in section I, B, 7, (e).

(e) SUMMARY

To save a considerable amount of repetition, section (d) above has been made to refer back to section (c) and that in turn to section (b). The following summary of all three sections will therefore be found useful, once their contents have been mastered:

	Self-Cleansing	*Self-Healing*	*Healing Others*
1	Perform at regular intervals	Perform when necessary	Perform when necessary
2	Light incense, three prostrations and (optional) offering mudrās		
3	Reflection on shortcomings, determination to do better	Reflection on sufferings of sentient beings and aspirations for their happiness	Aspiration for the health of the patient, visualised as present or actually present
4	Invocation to the Bodhisattva Kuan Yin.........................		
5	Visualisation of the ocean, moon and Bodhisattva..................		
6	Light enters own body, expelling karmic evils, which are swallowed by the sea-monsters, while one is uttering invocation or mantra	Light enters own body, expelling illness, which is swallowed by the sea-monsters, while one is uttering invocation or mantra	Light enters patient's body, expelling illness, which is swallowed by the sea-monsters, while one is uttering invocation or mantra
7	Rejoicing and gratitude on own behalf	Rejoicing and gratitude on own behalf	Rejoicing and gratitude on patient's behalf

8	Aspiration for the happiness of sentient beings	Aspiration for the health of sentient beings	Aspiration for the patient's health and well-being

9 Three prostrations and invocation of Kuan Yin....................

10 Three prostrations to the Triple Gem ....

(f) A STORY

Chang Jung, an erstwhile military commander in the forces of General Wu Pei-fu, being sickened by slaughter, had slipped away long before the General's downfall to become a wandering monk. It was his practice to walk from district to district in the southern part of his native Shantung province, where he gradually became known by sight to the local people. Having become a monk so late in life, he had not had to undergo a rigorous novitiate and was therefore careless in matters of detail. Every evening without fail, he used to recite Kuan Yin's Dhāranī of Great Compassion no less than one hundred and eight times, preferring to do so in the open air when the weather was clement. Now and then people saw rays of light playing around him and the more erudite recalled a passage in a sutra which runs: 'You should know that he is a treasure house of brilliance, for he is brightly illumined by the Tathāgatas [Buddhas]. You should know that he is a treasury of compassion, for he continually utters the Dhāranī of Great Compassion to rescue living beings.' It was generally believed that the old soldier was praying for the happy rebirth of the victims slaughtered in the battles of his unregenerate days.

Gradually, however, people's admiration for him began to wane. A rumour got about that, whenever he performed his practice out of doors, the grass close to where he had been sitting soon withered and that any small creatures that happened to be there, such as a colony of ants, would be found dead. Rocks and pebbles round about sometimes bore traces of odoriferous substances as though rotting corpses had been laid there. And so on. Much worse, if the weather had obliged him to perform his practice in a barn where he had chosen to pass the night, the floor was likely to be blotched with the same horrid substances, and sacks of grain that happened to be standing near might be blighted. As the people of the villages he visited from time to time did not like to refuse hospitality to such a holy man, they requested a learned Dharma Master to elucidate the cause of these strange happenings.

Greatly puzzled, the Dharma Master sought an opportunity to meet the former warrior. Courteously accosting him, he remarked: 'Venerable Sir, I have heard stories of lights shining around you when you are lost in contemplation. Wonderful indeed! I shall be grateful if you will relate to me in full your manner of cultivating the Way.'

This the old man did with pleasure.

'You actually see the bodies of those slain in battles long ago lying on the ground around you? When Kuan Yin Bodhisattva sheds her radiance upon them, the corpses exude evil substances to signify that, in response to your pious aspirations, those beings will be reborn in the Pure Land of Potala, or else born again in this world in happier circumstances than before? Great indeed is your merit!'

Chang Jung bowed his head as though unwilling to accept this praise, but a smile hovered on his lips.

'And what becomes of the evil substances that flow from their bodies?'

'*Becomes* of them?' queried the old man in considerable surprise. 'Why, nothing. Those corpses are, as Your Reverence knows well, creations of my mind during meditation. When I have completed one hundred and eight repetitions of the *dhāranī*, I withdraw my thoughts from those slaughtered beings and, of course, they vanish.'

The Dharma Master then explained that, during such visualisations, provision must be made for the disposal of discarded filth.

'Do you take me for a simpleton?' cried the old commander, laughing so heartily that the tears came to his eyes. 'How *can* one dispose of mentally created substances that do not actually exist?'

'*All* mind-created substances actually exist,' answered the Dharma Master reprovingly. 'What are your body and mine or this room where we now sit but mental creations? Pray come with me.'

Insisting that the incredulous Chang Jung walk back with him to the place where he had performed his practice on the previous evening, he pointed to some withered grass and to some rocks stained with a filthy substance from which even now a displeasing odour arose. Remorsefully the old man fell to his knees, albeit that the Dharma Master was his junior by many years, and cried: 'Alas, forgive me. This stupid old man is very much to blame. It was always dark by the time I completed my practice and, as I seldom stay in the same village for more than one night, these evidences of my folly quite escaped me. I beg Your Reverence to instruct me as to what it is proper for me to do.'

The Dharma Master complied most willingly. 'You must visualise the evil hosts of Yama hungrily gathering beneath the ground to feast upon what to them are the most delectable delicacies. In this way, you

pierce two targets with a single arrow by ensuring a happy rebirth for
the victims of the battles in which you had a share and, at the same
time, giving pleasure to the demon hosts. Nothing could be more
fitting, for demons love their pleasures just as men do, but it is not
always easy to satisfy them at no cost in human suffering. Hence the
beauty of a meditation practice that does good to all. It can have no
undesirable results whatsoever.' He then went on to explain that there
is no essential difference between the creations of individual minds
and those of Mind, that is to say, the entire universe; adding that there
is even less difference than usual when visualisation is performed by
an advanced yogin, such as Chang Jung, by reason of his unswerving
devotion to his fellow beings, had long since become.

'Please understand this clearly. You evoke the Bodhisattva Kuan
Yin in your mind. You see the lustrous rays that issue from her
forehead with your mind. You see the corpses of those slain in battle
with your mind. Yet do not suppose that they are unreal. The degree
of reality may differ somewhat from that of so-called solid objects, but
the difference is purely relative, not a difference in kind. If the
Compassionate Bodhisattva, her lustrous rays, the corpses of the slain
were altogether figments of your imagination, how could your pious
practices succeed in lightening the karmic load of those poor victims
slain by your men? Reality is not easy to define. Yet be sure that every
thought form, every dream, every vision is closer to objective reality
than you have hitherto supposed. What ordinary men call "objective
reality" appears quite otherwise to those who have learnt to see things
as they really are. In absolute terms, subject and object are not
different from each other. The thinker and the object of his thought
are most certainly NOT TWO!'

Not all the details of this curious story need be taken literally. Such
phenomena as the rays seen playing round the old monk during his
yogic practice are noted often enough for me to be unable to dismiss
them out of hand as allegory or fantasy. On the other hand, it is hard to
credit that failure to dispose mentally of visualised evil substances
could result in their leaving visible traces, withering the grass, killing
insects or blighting grain. I take this part of the story to indicate that,
should one mentally cast out pain or illness in the form of mind-
created evil substances and fail to dispose of them by a similar act of
mind, harmful psychic influences may linger round the place where
the healing or a similar practice is undertaken.

Appendices

The Dhāranī (or Mantra) of Great Compassion

Many devout Buddhists recite this *dhāranī* of Kuan Yin Bodhisattva a number of times every day of their lives. The Chinese or Japanese version may be substituted for the (reconstructed) Sanskrit version given in section II, B, 5, (d). The following Chinese text was kindly provided by the Institute for Advanced Studies of World Religions, New York. The romanisation complies with traditional rules for pronouncing Chinese characters when they have been used to transliterate Sanskrit syllables. (Note that the vowel Ē is to be pronounced like the vowel in the English word 'heed'.) Owing to the non-phonetic nature of the Chinese written language, the Chinese version is very far removed in sound from the original Sanskrit (which has unfortunately not survived). However, mispronunciation does not seem to affect the *dhāranī*'s marvellous efficacy, for it is recited in different parts of Asia with widely varying pronunciations, yet never ineffectively. Kuan Yin is, above all, compassionate! In uttering mantric syllables, one does not dwell upon (or even need to know) the verbal meaning, so this presents no problem.

NÁ MŌ HÅ LÅ DÁ NŌ DŌ LÅ YÁ YÁ　NÁ MŌ Ō LĒ YÁ　PŌ LU JĪ DĒ SŎ BŪ LÅ YÁ
PŌŌ TĒ SÅ DŎ PŌ YÁ　MŌ HŌ SÅ DŎ PŌ YÁ　MŌ HŌ JÅ LU NĒ JÅ YÁ　ĀN　SÅ
BU LÅ FÁ SHEH　SŌŌ DÁ NŌ DÁ SHÁ　NÁ MŌ SHI JĪ LĒ DŌ Ē MŌN Ō LĒ YÁ　PŌ LU
JĪ DĒ SŪ FU LÅ LÍN　TŌ PŌ　NÁ MŌ NŌ LÅ JĪN TSE　SHE LĒ MŌ HŌ BŪ DŎ SŎ MĒ
SÅ PŌ Ō TŌ DĒR SŌŌ PŌN　Ō SŬ YUÍN　SÅ PŌ SÅ DŎ NÁ MŌ PŌ SÅ DŎ NÁ MŌ PŌ CHÍA
MŌ FÁ DŬ DĒR　DÁ TZE TŌ　ĀN　Ō PŌ LU SHE LU CHÍA DĒ　JÅ LŌ DĒ　Ē SHE
LĒ　MŌ HŌ POO TE SÅ DŎ　SÅ PŌ SÅ PŌ　MŌ LÅ MŌ LÅ　MŌ SHE MŌ SHE　LĒ TŌ
YUÍN　JÜ LÜ JÜ LÜ JĪ MŌN　SÅ PŌ LÅ YÁ DE　MŌ HŌ FÁ SÅ YÁ DE
TŌ LÅ TŌ LÅ　SÅ LĒ NĒ　SÜ FŌ YÁ　DSŌ LÅ DSŌ LÅ　MŌ MŌ FÁ MŌ LÅ
MŌ DĒ LĒ　Ē SHE Ē SHE　SÜ NŌ SÜ NŌ　Ō LÅ SÜN FÙ LÅ SŎ LĒ　FÁ SŎ FÁ SÜN

FÚ LĂ SŌ YĂ 佛囉舍耶

HŌ LU HŌ LU MŌ LĂ 呼嚧呼嚧摩囉

HŌ LU HŌ LU SHĒ LĒ 呼嚧呼嚧醯利

SŌ LĂ SŌ LĂ 娑囉娑囉

SHĒ LĒ SHĪ LĒ 悉唎悉唎

SU LU SU LU 蘇嚧蘇嚧

POO TE YĂ POO TE YĂ 菩提夜菩提夜

POO TO YĂ POO TO YĂ 菩馱夜菩馱夜

MĒ DĒ LĒ YĂ 彌帝唎夜

NŌ LĂ JĪEN TSE 那囉謹墀

DĒ LĒ SĒ NĒ NŌ 地唎瑟尼那

PŌ YĂ MŌ NŌ 婆夜摩那

SŌ PŌ HŌ 娑婆訶

SHĪ TŌ YĂ 悉陀夜

SŌ PŌ HŌ 娑婆訶

MŌ HŌ SHĪ TŌ YĂ 摩訶悉陀夜

SŌ PŌ HŌ 娑婆訶

SHĪ TŌ YÜ YĒ 悉陀喻藝

SHĪ PŌ LĂ YĂ 室皤囉耶

SŌ PŌ HŌ 娑婆訶

NŌ LĂ JÏN TSĒ 那囉謹墀

SŌ PŌ HŌ 娑婆訶

MŌ LĂ NŌ LĂ 摩囉那囉

SŌ PŌ HŌ 娑婆訶

SŪ BU LĂ YĂ 悉囉僧

NŌ LĂ JÏEN TSE 阿穆佉耶

SŌ PŌ HŌ 娑婆訶

SHĪ LĂ SŪN O MŌ CHÏĂ YĂ 娑婆摩訶阿悉陀夜

SŌ PŌ HŌ 娑婆訶

JĀ JĪ LĂ O SHĪ TŌ YĂ 者吉囉阿悉陀夜

SŌ PŌ HŌ 娑婆訶

BŌ TŌ MŌ JĪ SHĪ TŌ YĂ 波陀摩羯悉陀夜

SŌ PŌ HŌ 娑婆訶

JÏEN TSE BU CHÏĂ LĂ YĂ 者吉囉阿悉陀夜

MŌ PŌ LĒ SÜN JĪ LĂ YĂ 摩婆利勝羯囉夜

SŌ PŌ HŌ 娑婆訶

NĂ MŌ HĂ LĂ DĂ NŌ DŌ LĂ YĂ YĂ 南無喝囉怛那哆囉夜耶

NÁ MŌ O LĒ YĂ 南無阿唎耶

BŌ LÔ JĪ DÉ 婆嚧吉帝

SŌ BU LĂ YĂ 爍皤囉夜

MĂN DŌO 漫都

SHĪ DÏEN DŌO 悉殿都

BU TŌ YĂ 跋陀耶

SŌ PŌ HŌ 娑婆訶

AN 唵

SŌ PŌ HŌ 娑婆訶

204 *Gateway to Wisdom*

The following alternative romanisation, kindly supplied by the Buddhist Text Translation Society, Gold Mountain Monastery, San Francisco, approximates to the present-day Northern Chinese pronunciation of the characters. (Note that syllables containing the vowel written WO, such as DWO and TWO, rhyme more or less with the English word 'roar', with the final r-sound suppressed as in southern England, but with just a suspicion of an oo-sound coming before the vowel proper. One could perhaps represent the sound thus – 'r°°oar'.)

DA BEI JOU GREAT COMPASSION MANTRA

NA MWO DA BEI GWAN SHR YIN PU SA (3 times)
Homage to the Greatly Compassionate Bodhisattva Who Contemplates the Sounds of the World

1) NA MWO HE LA DA NWO DWO LA YE YE
2) NA MWO E LI YE
3) PWO LU JYE DI SHAU BWO LA YE
4) PU TI SA TWO PE YE
5) MO HE SA DWO PE YE
6) MWO HE JYA LU NI JYA YE
7) NAN
8) SA PAN LA FA YE
9) SWO DA NWO DA SYE
10) NA MWO SYI JI LI TWO YI MENG E LI YE
11) PE LU JI DI SHR FWO LA LENG TWO PE
12) NA MWO NWO LA JIN CHR
13) SYI LI MWO HE PAN DWO SA MYE
14) SA PE E TWO DOU SHU PENG
15) E SHR YUN
16) SA PE SA DWO NA MWO PE SA DWO
17) NA MWO PE CHYE
18) MWO FA TE DOU
19) DA JR TWO
20) NAN
21) E PE LU SYI
22) LU JYA DI
23) JYA LA DI
24) YI SYI LI
25) MWO HE PU TI SA TWO
26) SA PE SA PE
27) MWO LA MWO LA
28) MWO SYI MWO SYI LI TWO YUN
29) JYU LU JYU LU JYE MENG
30) DU LU DU LU FA SHE YE DI
31) MWO HE FA SHE YE DI
32) TWO LA TWO LA

33) DI LI NI
34) SHR FWO LA YE
35) JE LA JE LA
36) MWO MWO FA MWO LA
37) MU DI LI
38) YI SYI YI SYI
39) SHR NWO SHR NWO
40) E LA SHEN FWO LA SHE LI
41) FA SHA FA SHEN
42) FWO LA SHE YE
43) HU LU HU LU MWO LA
44) HU LU HU LU SYI LI
45) SWO LA SWO LA
46) SYI LI SYI LI
47) SU LU SU LU
48) PU TI YE PU TI YE
49) PU TWO YE PU TWO YE
50) MI DI LI YE
51) NWO LA JIN CHR
52) DI LI SHAI NI NWO
53) PE YE MWO NWO
54) SWO PE HE
55) SYI TWO YE
56) SWO PE HE
57) MWO HE SYI TWO YE
58) SWO PE HE
59) SYI TWO YU YI
60) SHR PAN LA YE
61) SWO PE HE
62) NWO LA JIN CHR
63) SWO PE HE
64) MWO LA NWO LA
65) SWO PE HE
66) SYI LU SENG E MU CHYWE YE
67) SWO PE HE
68) SWO PE MWO HE E SYI TWO YE
69) SWO PE HE
70) JE JI LA E SYI TWO YE
71) SWO PE HE
72) BWO TWO MWO JYE SYI TWO YE
73) SWO PE HE
74) NWO LA JIN CHR PAN CHYE LA YE
75) SWO PE HE
76) MWO PE LI SHENG JYE LA YE
77) SWO PE HE
78) NA MWO HE LA DA NWO DWO LA YE YE
79) NA MWO E LI YE
80) PWO LU JYE DI

81) SHAU BWO LA YE
82) SWO PE HE
83) NAN
84) SYI DYAN DU
85) MAN DWO LA
86) BA TWO YE
87) SWO PE HE

The following romanised Japanese version of the same dhāranī was kindly sent to me by the Zen Centre, San Francisco. The vowels should be pronounced more or less in accordance with the international system of romanising foreign languages, which is based on Latin.

DAI HI SHIN DHĀRANĪ

NAMU KARA TAN NO TORA YA YA NAMU ORI YA BORYO
KI CHI SHIFU RA YA FUJI SATO BO YA MOKO SATO BO YA
MO KO KYA RUNI KYA YA EN SA HARA HA EI SHU TAN
NO TON SHA NAMU SHIKI RI TOI MO ORI YA BORYO KI CHI
SHIFU RA RIN TO BO NA MU NO RA KIN JI KI RI MO KO
HO DO SHA MI SA BO O TO JO SHU BEN O SHU IN SA BO
SA TO NO MO BO GYA MO HA TE CHO TO JI TO EN O BO
RYO KI RU GYA CHI KYA RYA CHI I KIRI MO KO FUJI SA
TO SA BO SA BO MO RA MO RA MO KI MO KI RI TO IN KU
RYO KU RYO KE MO TO RYO TO RYO HO JA YA CHI MO
KO HO JA YA CHI TO RA TO RA CHIRI NI SHIFU RA YA SHA
RO SHA RO MO MO HA MO RA HO CHI RI YU KI YU KI SHI NO
SHI NO ORA SAN FURA SHA RI HA ZA HA ZA FURA SHA
YA KU RYO KU RYO MO RA KU RYO KU RYO KI RI SHA RO
SHA RO SHI RI SHI RI SU RYO SU RYO FUJI YA FUJI YA
FUDO YA FUDO YA MI CHIRI YA NORA KIN JI CHIRI SHUNI
NO HOYA MONO SOMO KO SHIDO YA SOMO KO MOKO SHIDO
YA SOMO KO SHIDO YU KI SHIFU RA YA SOMO KO NORA
KIN JI SOMO KO MO RA NO RA SOMO KO SHIRA SU OMO
GYA YA SOMO KO SOBO MOKO SHIDO YA SOMO KO SHAKI
RA OSHI DO YA SOMO KO HODO MOGYA SHIDO YA SOMO
KO NORA KIN JI HA GYARA YA SOMO KO MO HORI SHIN
GYARA YA SOMO KO NAMU KARA TAN NO TORA YA YA
NAMU ORI YA BORYO KI CHI SHIFU RA YA SOMO KO SHITE
DO MODO RA HODO YA SO MO KO

*   *   *   *   *   *

JI HO SAN SHI I SHI FU
SHI SON BU SA MO KO SA
MO KO HO JA HO RO MI

APPENDIX 2

Text of the Heart Sutra (Prajñāpāramitāhṛdaya Sūtra)

My rendering and explanation of the sutra are given in section II, B, 5, (d). One may, of course, prefer to recite it in Chinese. The Institute for Advanced Studies of World Religions, New York, has kindly sent me the following Chinese text with a translation by Dr Garma C. C. Chang. His translation and mine agree well in all essentials, except that the names of the third and fourth aggregates or *skandhas* are rendered differently. The Buddhist scriptures contain so much learned disquisition on those two words (*saṃjñā* and *saṃskāra* in Sanskrit) that it is impossible to find English terms that give their full connotations; hence the Venerable Hsüan Hua, Abbot of Gold Mountain Monastery, explains them in yet another way:

	saṃjñā	*saṃskāra*
Abbot Hua	cognition	formation
Dr Chang	conceptions	impulses
Myself	perception	conditionings

We may take it that the Sanskrit terms each cover quite a number of meanings, including all those given here. Many Japanese translators render *saṃjñā* as 'thought', but I think this is an over-literal rendering of the Chinese character, rather than a good translation of the Sanskrit term. Japanese renderings of *saṃskāra* include 'volition', 'confection', 'imagination', 'activity' and 'active substance'.

PO JE PO LO MI TO HSIN CHING

般 若 波 羅 密 多 心 經

Hṛdaya Sūtra - Translated by Garma C. C. Chang

KUAN TZŬ TSAI P'U SA HSING SHEN PO JE PO LO MI TO SHIH

觀 自 在 菩 薩 行 深 般 若 沒 羅 密 多 時

When the Bodhisattva Avalokiteśvara was coursing in the deep Prajñāparamitā,

CHAO CHIEN WU YÜN CHIEH K'UNG TU YI CH'IEH

照 見 五 蘊 皆 空 度 一 切

he saw (intuitively) all the five skandhas are empty; thus he overcomes all

K'U EH SHEH LI TZU SEH PU YI K'UNG

苦 厄 舍 利 子 色 不 異 空

sufferings and ills. O Śariputra, form does not differ from Voidness, and

K'UNG PU YI SEH SEH CHI SHIH K'UNG K'UNG CHI SHIH SEH

空 不 異 色 色 即 是 空 空 即 是 色

Voidness does not differ from form. Form is Voidness, and Voidness is form;

SHOU HSIANG HSING SHIH YI FU JU SHIH

受 想 行 識 亦 復 如 是

likewise, the feelings, conceptions, impulses and consciousnesses.

SHEH LI TZU SHIH CHU FAH K'UNG HSIANG PU

舍 利 子 是 諸 法 空 相 不

O Śariputra, the characteristics of the Voidness of all dharmas are not

SHENG PU MIEH PU KOU PU CHING PU TSENG PU CHIEN

生 不 滅 不 垢 不 淨 不 增 不 減

arising, not ceasing; not defiled, not pure; not increasing, not decreasing.

SHIH KU K'UNG CHUNG WU SEH WU SHOU HSIANG HSING

是 故 空 中 無 色 無 受 想 行

Therefore in the Void there is no form, no feelings, conceptions, impulses,

SHIH WU YEN ER PI SHEH SHEN YI WU SEH SHENG

識 無 眼 耳 鼻 舌 身 意 無 色 聲

consciousnesses; no eye, ear, nose, tongue, body or mind; no form, sound,

HSIANG WEI CH'U FAH WU YEN CHIEH NAI CHIH WU

香 味 觸 法 無 眼 界 乃 至 無

smell, taste, touch or mind object; no eye elements, until we come to no

YI SHIH CHIEH WU WU MING YI WU WU MING CHIN

意 識 界 無 無 明 亦 無 無 明 盡

elements of consciousnesses; no ignorance and also no ending of ignorance,

NAI CHIH WU LAO SZŬ YI WU LAO SZŬ CHIN

乃 至 無 老 死 亦 無 老 死 盡

until we come to no old age and death and no ending of old age and death;

WU K'U CHI MIEH

無 苦 集 滅

no Truth of suffering, of the cause of suffering, of the cessation of suffering

TAO WU CHIH YI WU TEH

道 無 智 亦 無 得

and of the Path. There is no wisdom, and there is no attainment whatsoever.

YI WU SUO TEH KU P'U T'I SA TO YI PO JE

以 無 所 得 故 菩 提 薩 埵 依 般 若

Because there is no nothing to be attained, a Bodhisattva relying on Prajñā-

PO LO MI TO KU HSIN WU KUA AI WU KUA AI KU

波 羅 密 多 故 心 無 罣 礙 無 罣 礙 故

paramitā has no obstruction in his mind. Because there is no obstruction

WU YOU K'UNG PU YUAN LI TIEN TAO MENG HSIANG

無 有 恐 怖 遠 離 顛 倒 夢 想

he has no fear and he passes far beyond all confusions, imagination and
(finally)

CHIU CHING NIEH P'AN SAN SHIH CHU FU

究 竟 涅 槃 三 世 諸 佛

reaches the Ultimate Nirvāna. The Buddhas in the past, present and future,
also

YI PO JE PO LO MI TO KU TEH AH NOU TO LO SAN MIAO SAN P'U T'I

依 般 若 波 羅 密 多 故 得 阿 耨 多 羅 三 貌 三 菩 提

by relying on the Prajñāparamitā have attained the Supreme Enlightenment.

KU SHIH PO JE PO LO MI TO SHIH TA SHEN CHOU SHIH TA MING CHOU

故 知 般 若 波 羅 密 多 是 大 神 咒 是 大 明 咒

Therefore, the Prajñāparamitā is the great magic spell, is the great spell
of illumination,

SHIH WU SHANG CHOU SHIH WU TENG TENG CHOU NENG CH'U YI CH'IEH K'U

是 無 上 咒 是 無 等 等 咒 能 除 一 切 苦

is the supreme spell, is the unequalled spell which can truly protect one
from all sufferings

CHEN SHIH PU HSU KU SHUO PO JE PO LO MI TO CHOU CHI SHUO CHOU YUEH

真 實 不 虛 故 說 般 若 波 羅 密 多 咒 即 說 咒 曰

without fail.   Therefore he uttered the spell of Prajñāparamitā:

CHIEH TI CHIEH TI PO LO CHIEH TI PO LO SENG CHIEH TI   P'U T'I SA P'O HO

揭 諦   揭 諦 波 羅 揭 諦 波 羅 僧 揭 諦   菩 提 薩 婆 訶

Gaté,   Gaté,   Pāragaté,   Pārasamgaté,   Bodhi-svāhā.

The following is a romanised Japanese transliteration of the Heart
Sutra kindly supplied by the Zen Centre, San Francisco.

MA KA HAN NYA HA RA MIT TA SHIN GYO

KAN JI ZAI BO SATSU GYO JIN HAN NYA HA RA MIT TA JI
SHO KEN GO ON KAI KU DO IS SAI KU YAKU SHA RI SHI
SHIKI FU I KU KU FU I SHIKI SHIKI SOKU ZE KU KU SOKU
ZE SHIKI JU SO GYO SHIKI YAKU BU NYO ZE SHA RI SHI
ZE SHO HO KU SO FU SHO FU METSU FU KU FU JO FU ZO
FU GEN ZE KO KU CHU MU SHIKI MU JU SO GYO SHIKI MU
GEN NI BI ZES SHIN NI MU SKIKI SHO KO MI SOKU HO MU
GEN KAI NAI SHI MU I SHIKI KAI MU MU MYO YAKU MU
MU MYO JIN NAI SHI MU RO SHI YAKU MU RO SHI JIN MU
KU SHU METSU DO MU CHI YAKU MU TOKU I MU SHO TOK
KO BO DAI SAT TA E HAN NYA HA RA MIT TA KO SHIN MU
KE GE MU KE GE KO MU U KU FU ON RI IS SAI TEN DO MU
SO KU GYO NE HAN SAN ZE SHO BUTSU E HAN NYA HA RA
MIT TA KO TOKU A NOKU TA RA SAM MYAKU SAM BO DAI
KO CHI HAN NYA HA RA MI TA ZE DAI JIN SHU ZE DAI
MYO SHU ZE MU JO SHU ZE MU TO DO SHU NO JO IS SAI
KU SHIN JITSU FU KO KO SETSU HAN NYA HA RA MIT TA
SHU SOKU SETSU SHU WATSU GYA TE GYA TE HA RA GYA
TE HARA SO GYA TE BO JI SOWA KA HAN NYA SHIN GYO

*   *   *   *   *   *

JI HO SAN SHI I SHI FU
SHI SON BU SA MO KO SA
MO KO HO JA HO RO MI

APPENDIX 3

Text of a Poem from the Lotus Sutra

This famous description of the miraculous powers of the Bodhisattva Kuan Yin as the embodiment of invincible *mahā karunā* is recited many times every day by devout Buddhists. It should at least be read from time to time as an alternative (or, better still, an addition) to the Heart Sutra as part of the yogic rite described in section II, B, 5, (d):

> *World-Honoured Lord and Perfect One,*
> *I pray thee now declare*
> *Wherefore this holy Bodhisat*
> *Is known as Kuan Shih Yin?*
> *To this the Perfect One replied*
> *By uttering this song:*
>
> *The echoes of her holy deeds*
> *Resound throughout the world*
> *So vast and deep the vows she made*
> *When, after countless aeons*
> *Of serving hosts of Perfect Ones,*
> *She voiced her pure desire*
> *(To liberate afflicted beings).*
>
> *Now hearken to what came of it –*
> *To hear her name or see her form,*
> *Or fervently recite her name*
> *Delivers beings from every woe.*
>
> *Were you with murderous intent*
> *Thrust within a fiery furnace,*
> *One thought of Kuan Yin's saving power*
> *Would turn those flames to water!*
>
> *Were you adrift upon the sea*
> *With dragon-fish and fiends around you,*

One thought of Kuan Yin's saving power
Would spare you from the hungry waves.

Suppose from Mount Suméru's peak
Some enemy should cast you down,
One thought of Kuan Yin's saving power
And sun-like you would stand in space.

Were you pursued by evil men
And crushed against the Iron Mountain,
One thought of Kuan Yin's saving power
And not a hair would come to harm.

Were you amidst a band of thieves,
Their cruel knives now raised to slay,
One thought of Kuan Yin's saving power
And pity must restrain their blows.

Suppose the King now wroth with you,
The headsman's sword upraised to strike,
One thought of Kuan Yin's saving power
Would dash the sword to pieces.

Were you close pent by prison walls,
Your wrists and ankles bound with chains,
One thought of Kuan Yin's saving power
Would instantly procure release.

Had you imbibed some fatal draught
And lay now at the point of death,
One thought of Kuan Yin's saving power
Would nullify its poison.

Were you beset by raksa-fiends
Or noxious dragons, gibbering demons,
One thought of Kuan Yin's saving power
And none would dare offend you.

Did savage beasts press all around
With fearful fangs, ferocious claws,
One thought of Kuan Yin's saving power
Would send them helter-skelter.

Should serpents lie athwart your path
Exhaling noxious smoke and flame,
One thought of Kuan Yin's saving power
Would make them vanish fast as sound.

Should thunder roll and lightning flash,
Or fearsome rains come hissing down,
One thought of Kuan Yin's saving power
Would straightway lull the storm.

Though beings oppressed by karmic woes
Endure innumerable sorrows,
Kuan Yin's miraculous perception
Enables her to purge them all.

Imbued with supernatural power
And wise in using skilful means,
In every corner of the world
She manifests her countless forms.

No matter what black evils gather –
What hell-spawned demons, savage beasts,
What ills of birth, age, sickness, death,
Kuan Yin will one by one destroy them.

True Kuan Yin! Pure Kuan Yin!
Immeasurably wise Kuan Yin!
Merciful and filled with pity,
Ever longed-for and revered!

O Radiance spotless and effulgent!
O night-dispelling Sun of Wisdom!
O Vanquisher of storm and flame!
Your glory fills the world!

Your pity is a shield from lightning,
Your compassion forms a wondrous cloud
Which, raining down the Dharma-nectar,
Extinguishes the flames of woe.

To those enmeshed in litigation
Or trembling in the midst of hosts
There comes the thought of Kuan Yin's power,
Whereat all hatred is dispersed.

The mysterious sound of Kuan Yin's name
Is holy like the ocean's thunder –
No other like it in the world!
And therefore should we speak it often.

Call upon it, never doubting,
Kuan Shih Yin— sound pure and holy;
To those who stand in mortal fear
A never-wavering support.

To the perfection of her merits,
To the compassion in her glance,
To the infinitude of her blessings,
Worshipping, we bow our heads!